The Doctor Is IN

*Answering Your Questions About
How to Survive Caregiving*

CHERYL E. WOODSON, MD, FACP, AGSF, CHCQM
Family Caregiver, Geriatrician

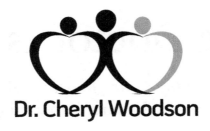

Dr. Cheryl Woodson

Category: Non-Fiction/Self-Help-Caregiving/Geriatrics

ISBN: 978-0-9967809-1-9   Paperback
ISBN: 978-0-9967809-4-0   eBook

Second Edition, November 2021.

The Five Keys to Caregiver Survival

n my other caregiver resource, *To Survive Caregiving: A Daughter's Experience, A Doctor's Advice*, I explain the Five Keys to Caregiver Survival. Since I refer to them in the text, I list them here for your convenience. You may also get a free copy by signing into my website: www.drcherylwoodson.com.

1. **Don't Stick Your Head in the Sand**
   According to folklore, ostriches do this because they believe danger can't see them if they can't see danger. However, ostriches get their backsides shot off all the time That's why there are ostrich burgers in specialty grocery stores. If you put your head in the sand, you present a bigger target. *Find out if you need help.*

2. **Take the "S" off Your Chest or Step Away from the Kryptonite**
   You are not *Supercaregiver!*
   You do need help.

3. **"Don't Ask, Don't Tell" Won't Work**
   Tell people you need help.

4. **If You Don't Want to Drive All the Time, Take Your Hands Off the Steering Wheel**
   Let people help.

5. **Put Your Mask on First**
   This is what flight attendants tell you to do when there is an in-flight emergency. *You can't take care of them if you don't take care of you.*

TABLE OF CONTENTS

INTRODUCTION

You Asked; I Answered

I wrote *The Doctor is IN* as a companion book for the second edition of *To Survive Caregiving: A Daughter's Experience, A Doctor's Advice* (which is also available at your bookseller, right now).

I have traveled around the country to give presentations about family caregiving, professional eldercare, geriatrics, healthcare public policy, the aging workforce, understanding managed care, and how to *LIVE OUT LOUD AND AGE EXCELLENTLY!* After each presentation, there were lively Q and A sessions where caregivers said I gave information they hadn't heard anywhere else. Though I understood that their questions deserved more thoughtful and complete answer than I could offer in fifteen-minute a Q and A session, as I started the second edition of *To Survive Caregiving*, I realized the questions were beyond the scope of that book too. *The Doctor Is IN* addresses many of these questions and shares strategies I recommended to families in more than thirty years of practice in Geriatric Medicine. The book also shares wisdom from many of the caregivers I met in those thirty years and from my own experience caring for my mom.

I don't know how to handle any subject except head-on. Some topics may feel uncomfortable but please stay with me while we walk through them. If we don't deal with these issues, they deal with us anyway. They simmer inside us until they putrefy our spirits, sap our energy, and erode our joy.

In *The Doctor is IN*, I suggest ways to think about and manage many of these challenges, including how to:

- Work with overly demanding seniors
- Meet the challenge of seniors who mismanage money, with special attention to seniors who support younger adults who should take responsibility for themselves
- Decide whether a senior should live with an adult child
- Recognize and avoid elder abuse and neglect and

- Address the physical intimacy challenges of people whose spouses have Alzheimer's disease.

One chapter delves into the danger of using caregiving to meet our needs instead of developing healthy activities and relationships. Another chapter shows what happens when you allow stress to ravage your body. There are also resources to help you *LIVE OUT LOUD AND AGE EXCELLENTLY!* as you avoid the health challenges your seniors face. Another chapter empowers you to advocate for your loved ones in the new healthcare system. My coach, Monique Caradine-Kitchens, requested the chapter, *"Prepare to Care,"* for the twenty-, thirty-, and forty-year-olds who worry about future caregiving. The recommendations will help pre-caregivers who are concerned about the future as well as the people who have to prepare to care again tomorrow.

Many caregivers asked for advice about how to reorient themselves once the season of caregiving has passed. For them, I interviewed several recovering caregivers for the chapter, *"Life After Caregiving."*

After addressing specific caregiver questions, I added a few chapters to shed light on some covert dangers in caregiving and strengthen your armor against them. There is also a special chapter from my Care Warriors, seasoned caregivers that I met in my medical practice who have specific, practical and essential wisdom to help you get through.

A Few Housekeeping Issues

Like *To Survive Caregiving, The Doctor is IN* shares stories that illustrate the struggles of caregivers in my medical practice or problems I faced in my own caregiving. I separate these stories from the rest of the text with asterisks (*****). To be clearer and more concise, in some chapters, I present composites of several family stories. However, the situations, challenges, and solutions are *real*. Although some individuals gave me permission to use their names, I changed other names and identifying characteristics to protect seniors' and caregivers' privacy. I picked the substitute names at random, without any intention of referring to real persons, living or dead. Any similarity to such persons is entirely coincidental.

To avoid the cumbersome phrases, "his or hers," "he or she," and "him or her," unless the text refers to a specific person, or a situation that affects men and women differently, I will say "they" or I will alternate pronouns.

I Know There's a Lot of Information

These chapters are responses to questions from real caregivers. Many told me this information is new to them and they would not have known where to find it. Take your time. You don't have to digest everything at once. Read at your own pace and feel free to jump around and read topics as you need them. Even if you read straight through, you will probably find that you'll re-read the information-dense sections several times. No matter how you use this resource, you will find information that comforts, encourages, and prepares you to take care of your seniors and yourself.

Caregiving Is a Team Sport

I rely on your feedback to ensure that I continue to give the most effective help. Contact me via www.drcherylwoodson.com to ask questions, give comments, and share your wisdom. I'm sorry I can't acknowledge every comment. I will incorporate your ideas into topics for future blog posts and podcasts, "Straight Talk with Dr. Cheryl". I would also love to meet you at a presentation. Visit my website, www.drcherylwoodson.com, for information about of upcoming events and publications and to schedule an interview or seminar.

Thank you.
—CW

CHAPTER 1

Are You Too Stressed to Be Blessed? *Stress Can Kill You!*

D o you feel like you have so much going on that you can't take a breath, get a break, or even think straight? Stress is not an illusion, a character flaw, or a state of mind. Stress causes significant emotional and physical problems for the caregiver and the senior.

Stress is a Normal, Protective Reaction to Immediate Danger

The stress response developed in all animals as a form of protection and survival. It is a fight, flight, or freeze instinct: defend, run away, or be very still and hope the danger will not see you as it passes by.

When you need to run from a predator, your body puts out stress hormones that increase your breathing, heart rate, and blood pressure. This stress reaction delivers more blood and oxygen to your muscles so you can stand and fight, run away, or be ready to do either if you freeze first and need to switch gears. This process shunts blood away from the stomach and other internal organs that do not participate in the emergency response. These body systems stay on high alert until the danger passes. Then, the level of stress hormones is supposed to decrease. Bodily functions are supposed to go back to a normal resting state.

Unfortunately, you can't fight your job, family, financial problems, or an unsafe neighborhood; most of us can't run away from these realities, either. Although we may freeze and put up with stressful circumstances, these life challenges don't go away. Our bodies stay on alert, and our stress-hormones never return to the lower, resting levels. This causes problems in many parts of the body.[1, 2]

Stress Kills! Your Brain Can't Think, and
Your Body Can't Work Well Under Constant Stress.

Research has shown that long-term stress damages our brains. Scientists studied the brains of animals that live in social structures similar to humans and found that constantly high stress hormone levels cause brain cells to shrink. This damage is concentrated in the frontal lobes, where complex thinking begins. There is also shrinkage in the hippocampus, a structure deep in the brain that is important for memory.[3]

These thinking and memory centers slow down while activity increases in the amygdala, another deep brain structure that influences anger and anxiety. The amygdala is also important in experiencing pleasure and may have a role in overeating and other addictions.[4] Eldercare, childcare, work, and other responsibilities leave many caregivers with little time to sleep. High levels of stress hormones can interfere with the normal sleep cycle and ruin the sleep they do get. Sleep deprivation can amplify the effects of stress, increasing irritability, fatigue, poor concentration, and poor judgment.[5,6]

These brain changes can lead caregivers to make mistakes in giving medicines, miss appointments, confuse treatment schedules, and have a higher risk of other kinds of accidents. These changes may also explain why some caregivers just can't stop snapping at everybody while others succumb to paralyzing worry, depression, drugs, or alcohol. Others just disconnect and go numb. They've pickled their brains in stress hormones!

Persistently high blood pressure affects the heart and blood vessels, increasing the risk of heart disease and stroke. This jazzed-up hormonal state can also interfere with blood sugar levels and worsen the complications of diabetes. High levels of stress hormones can increase appetite and change the way our bodies store fat. This causes weight gain that increases the risk of heart disease, diabetes, and stroke. Stress damages the immune system by decreasing the activity of white blood cells that fight infections and cancer.[7] Stress can also cause a queasy stomach, constipation, and belly pain which can make people believe that their life is no longer worth living.

Can We Be Easier On Ourselves?

A lot of stress is internal and has more to do with the way we have learned to respond to a situation than the situation itself. Pastor Mike Russell of Jubilee Faith Community in Country Club Hills, IL explained it to me by paraphrasing an old Buddhist saying.

"Pain [life-challenge] is mandatory; suffering is optional."

We can feel so overwhelmed by stress that we launch into frantic behavior without thinking. This automatic reaction compounds our stress and seldom works, anyway.

Behavioral health professionals describe post-traumatic stress disorder (PTSD) in people who have experienced, witnessed, or otherwise encountered war, violence, abuse, or other forms of trauma.[8] When people who live with PTSD encounter a sound, sight, smell, situation, or even a thought that reminds them of the original trauma, they experience the same mental and bodily stress reactions as when it first happened. I believe people can also suffer from what I've learned to call *pre-traumatic stress*. They go into full stress-mode worrying about what might happen in the future.

How to Manage Stress

Wouldn't we all like to relieve our stress on the beach in Hawaii? Though that would be nice, stress-management doesn't have to be fancy, time-consuming, or expensive. Any kind of regular exercise will help manage stress, and it does not always require expensive equipment, classes, or gym memberships. Walking, dancing, bowling, swimming, skating, stretching, anything you enjoy will do. Mindfulness is an approach to stress- management that encourages us to acknowledge and respect our thoughts, emotions, and how our bodies feel at the present moment. In addition to working with a trained behavioral health therapist, you can explore several techniques including deep breathing, meditation, yoga, or Reiki (a Japanese form of energy-healing designed to reduce stress and promote wellness). Churches, park districts, and community colleges, offer affordable classes. There are also virtual sessions online and even apps for your phone.

It can be equally effective to set aside regular times for activities and people you enjoy or to just relax and do nothing. You *do* have time. You have every minute God has given you. You *can* learn how to invest that time in ways that help manage your stress. If you don't learn how to protect time for yourself, you can find yourself using all of Eternity sooner than you would like. One of the fifty-eight-year-old caregivers in my practice dropped dead and left two eighty-year-olds behind. She knew to the last pill when the seniors needed new prescriptions, but she hadn't taken time to protect her own health and joy.

It is also important to figure out exactly why you are stressed and learn to address any underlying issues you haven't noticed.

>*>*>*>*>*>*>*>*>*>*>*>*>*>*

Mrs. Allen was bouncing off the walls. She had primary responsibility for her mother-in-law, Mamie, who had mild dementia. Mother Mamie lived alone though she needed daily setup and supervision for her medicines and assistance with housekeeping, meals, and transportation for shopping, hair and doctor appointments. Mrs. Allen took Mother Mamie out to lunch almost every day and attended a weekly dance class with her. They had a day to attend seminars at the library and another day each week to ride the train downtown to one of the museums. On other days, Mrs. Allen took Mother Mamie grocery shopping or let her help with laundry and other chores for both households.

At every office visit, Mrs. Allen said the situation was "okay," until her own mother planned to visit from out of state.

"I have to paint my kitchen," Mrs. Allen said as she wrung her hands and paced in my office. "How am I going to paint my kitchen when I don't have anybody to stay with Mother Mamie? She does so much better when she keeps to her usual routine."

Mrs. Allen was in a frenzy until we started brainstorming about how she could carve out time to paint the kitchen. She shot down every suggestion until I asked, "Why do you have to paint the kitchen?"

She looked at me as if she had never considered that question.

>*>*>*>*>*>*>*>*>*>*>*>*>*>*

Do "the Work" by Byron Katie

Author Byron Katie teaches a stress-busting, misery-easing philosophy called "The Work." She says,

> *"The Work is a simple, yet powerful inquiry that teaches you to question and identify the thoughts that cause all the suffering in the world. It's a way to understand what's hurting you and to address the cause of your problems with clarity."* [9]

According to The Work, there are two kinds of "truths" that control behavior: the ones you are willing to question and others that you will not challenge because you "know" they are the T-R-U-T-H. You can tell the type of "truth" that is in control because the ones you refuse to question cause the most emotional pain. These unquestionable truths hurt because of the amount of energy we invest to avoid or protect beliefs we are afraid to confront. Byron Katie says we must confront these beliefs before we can, *"Find resolution, even happiness, in situations that were once debilitating."* (10)

Instead of refusing to question, we can work on "loving what is" (11) and embrace reality. This frees us to find ways to experience joy instead of stress. Before we rush to respond to a situation in the same old, stressful way, The Work says we should ask these four questions. I presented them to Mrs. Allen (with my own explanations).

1) **Is this true?**
   Will someone die, end up in the hospital, or go bankrupt if you don't paint the kitchen?

2) **How do you know it's true?**
   Although you may fear or believe this is true, what is the *objective* evidence that you need to paint? For example, the last time your mother came to visit, did she walk straight into your kitchen, put her hands on her hips, and say, "Well, at least you could have painted?" Although some mother-daughter relationships include this type of rudeness, Mrs. Allen agreed that she had a loving relationship with her mother. There was neither history nor other evidence to justify her worry.

3) **Who would you be if you didn't need it to be true?**
   Caregivers often forget to think about how they feel or understand that they don't deserve to suffer the way they do. I always ask, "Why do you need to do this to yourself? Why do you need to add this extra stress?" You don't deserve the stress. "How would your life change if you didn't believe this? Might you be able to feel better?"

4) **Is there any good reason to keep believing this?**
   I tell caregivers that a *good* reason is one that creates love, support, and validation for YOU.

****

After Mrs. Allen answered these questions, she admitted that she didn't *need* to paint. She was exhausted by being her mother-in-law's sole caregiver, and she was upset because there was no time for herself. Mrs. Allen had also been afraid her husband would be critical if she told him the situation was unfair. Things came to a head because Mrs. Allen didn't want her eighty-year-old mother to make a 300-mile drive by herself. Mrs. Allen also wanted some alone-time with her mom during the visit. She wanted to fly out, enjoy the drive with her mother, show Mom around the city, and fly her mother back home.

Mrs. Allen and I scheduled a family conference with her husband and his siblings to tell them she was taking time off to be with *her* mother. The siblings would have to cover *their* mother for two weeks and think about other care options for the long-term.

After her mother went home, Mrs. Allen's husband and his family admitted they'd had no idea how hard Mrs. Allen worked to take care of their mother. They agreed to move Mother Mamie into an assisted-living community for people with memory loss. Mrs. Allen still takes her mother-in-law to dance class one day each week and out to lunch another day. She calls Mother Mamie frequently, takes her to the doctor, and participates in family activities at the facility when she can. Mrs. Allen also goes to the gym, enjoys a book club with friends, and takes a pottery class. She is also much less stressed.

****

Sometimes, being stressed about a seemingly simple thing is a sign of bigger, more complicated problems that you haven't been able (or willing) to address. Your answers to the four "WORK" questions can help you move minor issues that don't need action and reveal the challenges that do. When the circumstances require action, these questions let you take a breath and step away for a moment. This little break can decrease the negative impact of stress. When you settle yourself and think more clearly, you may make better decisions.

Caregivers need clear heads for one the most difficult decisions, which I describe in the next chapter: should you and your senior should share a home?

CHAPTER 2

Should Dad Move in with Us?
What Should We Consider?

It can be a blessing when seniors and their adult children choose to live together. The situation allows many grateful caregivers to support parents who supported them. It can also create opportunities for meaningful intergenerational sharing. For example, Grandma passes wisdom, and the kids teach her about computers. In other cases, seniors demand to move into an adult child's home, or adult children make the demands. Whether families see this choice as a blessing or a stressor, the situation can disrupt the lives of everyone involved. The key to making a decision that works for everyone is *honest* consideration of the wishes and needs of *all* parties. This requires clear communication, flexibility, and compromise.

****

Mrs. Vernon is a corporate attorney and her husband is the master chef at an elite restaurant. They had been married more than twenty years and had decided not to have children. The Vernons had built their home as a peaceful refuge on three acres outside the city. The first-floor master suite offered a spa-like oasis. A winding grand staircase led to other bedrooms that they used for offices, a library, and a music room. Every night, they would retreat from their hectic professional lives to cook gourmet meals together, read, listened to jazz or classical music, and play chess or backgammon as they sipped fine wine. They also traveled frequently, enjoying spontaneous weekend getaways and well-planned, long vacations.

Mrs. Vernon's mother and stepfather, Gary, lived several states away. Although Mrs. Vernon did not see her mom often, they spoke on the phone several times every week. When her mother died, Gary began to call Mrs. Vernon almost every night to complain about his health, the repairs needed on his mobile home, and everything else.

Mrs. Vernon and her husband visited Gary several times and always came back completely stressed out because his life was very different from theirs. Gary used a loud and colorful collection of swear words; he liked vintage country music, smoked cigars, and drank lots of straight bourbon. When they were at home, the Vernons spent many a previously peaceful evening either enduring exhausting, one-sided cursing, complaining phone sessions with Gary, or dreading his calls. They panicked when he started talking about moving in with them.

Mr. and Mrs. Vernon had several thoughtful discussions about a new living situation. They knew Gary was lonely; he had lost not only his wife but also many of the friends they had shared. Many of his Army buddies and his brother had passed on, and he was estranged from his adult children and their families. The Vernons knew they had more than enough space. The stairs would be a problem because of Gary's arthritis, and the couple did not relish the idea of giving up their master suite. Though they wanted to help, they knew their lifestyle and Gary's were incompatible.

The Vernons decided to suggest that Gary move to their city, into a nearby senior community with lots of amenities and activities. The couple hired a professional eldercare consultant to handle urgent needs and to be on call when they travel. They talk to Gary every few days. They also share weekly outings with him though they often have to schedule these activities around his poker tournaments. The Vernons continue to have peaceful evenings, and everyone is satisfied with the compromise.

****

When caregivers decide to move seniors into their homes, they expect to change the environment to make it accessible, comfortable, and safe for the senior's level of independence. Unfortunately, they often overlook several other factors critical to a successful move.

Routine

This is the time to get out the family organizational calendar. Things can get very tense when your choir rehearsal or your teenager's basketball practice conflicts with Mom's poker night and there's only one available driver. What happens when Dad insists on watching his favorite talk show in the middle of your book club meeting?

If the senior reacts well to change, wonderful. If not, don't give in to thoughts of "why-do-I-have-to-put-up-with-this-in-my-own-house?" That will just scuttle the plan. Everyone's priorities are important, and everyone deserves respect. Everybody will also have to be flexible. Blending lives will take creativity and compromise. Sit down and get potential (or real) conflicts and resentments out on the table. Don't get stuck nursing and rehearsing the grievances; try to figure out what *can* work. Can you, your son, and your Mom rotate carpooling with other people who participate in their respective activities? Can you use rideshare resources? Can your book club meet at the public library or coffee shop while Dad watches his show? Can you rotate the meeting among members, or set up a television for Dad in another room?

Even though compromise is key, in my experience, many caregivers completely give up what's important to them to make their seniors comfortable. It is important not to do this because it breeds resentment and can lead to irritability or depression. If you love to play pool, play pool. You can develop a plan that works for everyone.

Respite for You and for Your Senior

Respite is a break from responsibility. Don't wait until you break to get a break. Plan regular respite time so you have something to look forward to. If your senior is disabled, you *should not* be on duty 24/7/365 just because you live in the same house. I realize that families often make the decision to co-habitate because of strained finances but as much as you can, continue to make regular use of adult day centers and in-home care services. Also, accept help from friends and recruit support from your family and community. Even if the senior is not disabled, you are not solely responsible for her activities and entertainment. Insist on your "me" time and encourage your senior to participate in independent activities to the level of her interests and abilities.

Just as you are not always on call for your senior, you should not ignore the senior's priorities for your convenience. Her time, needs, and interests are equally valuable. While everyone should be included in family routines and responsibilities, you should not expect seniors to babysit, cook, or provide other services just because they are at home or because you think they have nothing else to do. Instead of taking the senior's availability for granted, respect his time and get permission before you assign a task. Discuss and agree about responsibilities and priorities when you plan the move, always have back up resources, and give adequate notice for schedule changes.

Remember, Your Senior Is an Adult

In trying to care for an older adult, families can be overbearing and violate the senior's well-earned independence.

****

Mrs. Yarborough is an independent eighty-seven-year-old woman who took out her trash on a snowy day, fell, and broke her knee. After the surgery, she went to a skilled nursing facility for short-term physical therapy.

The senior was deeply committed to her recovery. In the nursing home, she followed the physical therapists' instructions and did additional exercises on her own several times each day. The therapists were amazed at her progress and agreed to an early discharge.

Though Mrs. Yarborough wanted to go home, her son, David and his wife, Carol, insisted she come to their house. They pestered the senior to take more naps and refused to buy the ice cream bars she loved. Mrs. Yarborough stuck to her rigorous exercise schedule even though her son and daughter-in-law were convinced that she was "doing too much." Against medical advice, her son told the physical therapist that his mother would attend outpatient sessions only once rather than three times per week. David and Carol hired a caregiver, but Mrs. Yarborough almost ran her companion ragged by continually increasing the length of her walks. Once, I saw the caregiver sitting in a food court, looking exhausted. She said Mrs. Yarborough was on her fourth trip around the mall.

Though Mrs. Yarborough felt ready to return to her home, the younger Yarboroughs decided she should live with them permanently. There were loud arguments daily. Everyone was miserable until the furious senior arranged a conference with her family in my office. Even though the physical therapist and I assured David and Carol that Mrs. Yarborough was doing well, the younger Yarboroughs did not give in.

I ordered a driving assessment, which demonstrated that Mrs. Yarborough was a safe driver. Mental status testing found that she was capable of making sound decisions. She was physically capable of carrying out those decisions, and I supported her choice to return to her home. I also cleared her to have a couple of ice cream bars per week. To put the family's mind at ease, I recommended that Mrs. Yarborough compromise and agree to have the companion at her house a few hours each day. The worker would accompany her on errands and help with shopping, cooking, and housekeeping.

Two years later, after I retired from practice, I ran into Mrs. Yarborough in the women's locker room at a community health and wellness center. She was excited about taking a senior water aerobics class. Her companion was sitting in the waiting area, drinking a smoothie.

****

As much as you would like to protect your seniors, you can't disregard what is important to them. Yes, it is your home but when they come to live with you, it's their home too. Don't be ageist and assume that older adults *should* be disabled. Neither should you confuse being helpful with the need to control. Instead of rejecting the seniors' wishes out of hand, ask whether it is safe for the senior to do what she wants to do. Your senior's doctor should be able to provide what I call the **Level of Care Prescription** or LOCRx. Chapter Three: *When the Doctor Says It is Not Safe for the Senior To… Balance Independence and Safety*, fully describes LOCRx™. Briefly, this term describes recommendations that health professionals make after they review test results. The information tells families how much care the senior needs (if any) and reveals whether the older adult's wishes are realistic or not. Then professionals use the LOCRx to recommend the safest place for the senior to live. If seniors are physically and mentally capable and you intend to share living space, you need to find ways to compromise.

You Are Also an Adult

If your parent lives with you and still sees you as a child, life can deteriorate into the kinds of battles you had when you were a teenager. You can feel threatened, revert to old behaviors, and respond with whining or anger as if you were still a child. To avoid this, remember that among adults, *respect does not equal obedience.* Whether your seniors accept it or not, you *are* an adult. You need to accept it too.

Hear with your "Big-Kid" Ears. *No Threat? No Fight*

As an adult, you have full and final authority over your life, your children, your money, and other life decisions. Once you realize your parents have no real power, you will see there is no threat. Then, the need to fight can fade away.

I know it won't be easy. This can be an especially big problem when your relationship with the senior has been difficult. Conditional love, undermining or mean statements, and disapproval can really hurt.

****

My mother created me. She was brilliant and she felt frustrated by the barriers that blocked the dreams of so many young Black women in North Philadelphia in the 1940s. I would not be the woman I am if Mother's frustration had not fueled her determination that my brother and I would succeed despite *any* obstacles.

It was hard for Mother to step out of that coaching role. Even after I had a successful career, a lovely home, and a growing family, she always acted as if she thought, "Oh, you didn't do what I suggested? You must not have *heard* me." She would start with "helpful" comments that escalated to disapproval and even ridicule when I didn't change my plans. Once, she even tried to interfere.

As I grew up, Mother had been my advocate, mentor, anchor, and the standard against which I measured myself. It hurt so much that it seemed she didn't trust me, didn't believe I was capable, and was *disappointed* in me. With time and support, I learned to trust *myself*. Instead of going into battle, I would say something like:

> "Mother, I understand you believe that's what I should do, and I appreciate how much you care. I considered what you said and decided to do it another way."

At first, she would turn up the heat with even more painful disapproval and every time, it was hard not to go into battle. However, as I continued to trust myself, I could respect her without explaining, defending, or arguing. I would thank her and do what I had decided to do. Eventually, Mother backed down. She wasn't happy about it, but she backed down.

****

Most of us learn knee-jerk reactions to parental disapproval in childhood, and we perfect those reactions over decades. Even so, you are no longer eight years old. You're thirty-eight, forty-eight, fifty-eight, even sixty-eight, right? You *are* an adult. I know your parents' comments really hurt. However, when you learn to hear them with "big-kid" ears, you can avoid or de-escalate these battles by always behaving like an adult. I know it hurts and I don't pretend that you won't have these discussions again and again. You may need counseling to help you learn to interrupt the cycle of ineffective, old reactions. That's okay. Do what you have to do to avoid descending into defensive arguments; they only increase your stress.

It's harder to hear with "big-kid" ears and behave like an adult when you need the older person's money. It is important that you...

Maintain Everyone's Financial Independence

Many families base the decision to live together on improving *everyone's* finances. Even so, caregivers should not expect to use seniors' assets for their own needs or for the needs of their families. Even if you provide financial support to your senior, keep her finances separate from your own. The best way to do this is with a written agreement that documents negotiated financial responsibilities (like who will pay which household expenses) as you would with a roommate. Keep strict accounts of all bills and document clearly how you use seniors' pension funds, Social Security, other income, and your own money for the household and other expenses on the senior's behalf. This strategy maintains the boundaries you place on the senior's access to your money and decreases the risk that you will slip into the crime of financial exploitation. (See Chapter Four: *When Seniors Mismanage or Struggle with Money* and the section on "Financial Exploitation" in Chapter Nine: *Elder Mistreatment-Abuse and Neglect*).

Sanctuary

All members of the household deserve space and time to call their own. Be mindful of privacy issues for the senior, teenagers, children, and other members of the household. Don't forget sanctuary for yourself. The ability to retreat to a peaceful spot can mean the difference between family harmony and painful strife. Since most families don't have the luxury of a mansion with separate wings, schedule use of shared spaces and make sure everyone has alone time when they need it.

Accept Your Discomfort and Doubts; Respect Your Wishes

If in your heart, you don't *want* to move a senior into your home, don't do it. You don't need a specific reason. It's enough that you don't want to. Don't say what you think people want to hear or do what you believe they expect. You deserve your space and the senior deserves to feel welcome and at home.

If you cannot compromise or agree on a living situation that works well for everyone, a counselor can help you be clear and honest about what you need and avoid acting out of guilt. Ask your doctor for a referral to a social service professional who can help you explore other residential options.

The Same Considerations Apply if You Move into The Senior's Home

Once you decide to share a living space, everyone should feel at home. This will not work if anyone believes, "You're in my house; you're here to serve me," or "I gave up everything to move in here to take care of you; you should be grateful." You should not have to give up everything, nor should you expect the senior to do so. Both parties should communicate as *adults* and respect each other's needs, wishes, and privacy. Everyone must be prepared to plan and compromise about the use of space, schedules, and resources. Again, careful documentation and separation of finances is critical to avoiding financial exploitation on either side.

Neither you nor the senior should feel like a captive babysitter, cook, maid, or chauffeur. There must be clear communication on responsibility for chores, bills, and transportation. Even though you live there, you should not be on call 24 hours every day. It is also important to continue to reach for family and community resources to avoid caregiver burnout.

Of course, many adult children and their parents are thrilled to share a residence. Please understand that no matter how cordial the relationship or how wonderful everyone finds the situation, there will be times when you'll wish you had your own space. That's okay. Give yourself a break. Anticipate uncomfortable feelings; make sure you have your schedules, sanctuary, and respite resources in place so everyone can take a step away and take care of themselves. This approach will help everyone make better decisions about what is the safest, most appropriate, and most respectful situation for all.

CHAPTER 3

When the Doctor Says It's Not Safe for Your Loved One to... *Balance Independence and Safety with the Level of Care Prescription (LOCRx)*

One of the biggest challenges caregivers face is how to keep seniors safe without unnecessary restrictions. I have developed the concept, The Level of Care Prescription (LOCRx), to describe a care-planning process that shows families how the senior's medical conditions affect their abilities. This information can resolve confusion about whether it is safe for the senior to do what she wants to do. It also relieves tension when a family's expectations are beyond a senior's ability. Instead of feeling frustrated that the senior is "stubborn," "faking," "lazy," or "just trying to get on my nerves," these families can accept the elder's limitations.

The Level of Care Prescription (LOCRx)

Ten questions allow health professionals to tailor a care plan to your senior's needs.

The first five questions define the illness:

- What is wrong? (What are the senior's problems?)
- Why is it wrong? (The illnesses that cause those problems)
- How much is fixable?
- How do we fix the fixable issues?
- What do we do with the conditions we can't fix?

The second five questions develop the care plan:

- What type(s) of care does the senior need?
  (Household help or medical care?)
- How much care does she need?
  (Are the tasks simple or complicated?)
- How often does he need the care?
  (Daily, weekly, 4x a day?)
- How long will she need the care?
  (Weeks, months, a lifetime?)
- How much education should the caregiver have?
  (Can the grandson perform the task, or does the senior need a registered nurse?)

A specialized team can perform a **comprehensive geriatrics assessment** to develop the LOCRx. This team includes geriatricians (physicians who specialize in the care of older adults), nurses, therapists in rehabilitation and behavioral health services, and social workers. Some teams also include pharmacists, nutritionists, community service workers, and clergy.

This geriatrics assessment goes beyond the traditional medical examination that focuses on the senior's physical condition. It also tests brain function and the level of independence for mobility, performing daily tasks for personal care, and other responsibilities. The team also reviews the senior's prescriptions and over-the-counter medicines to remove unnecessary drugs and ensure that all treatments are *gero-friendly* (appropriate for a senior's age, health goals, and overall condition).

If there is a disability, the team will recommend treatments, equipment, environmental or behavioral changes to support the senior and allow as much independence as possible. The social service members of the geriatrics team review the LOCRx and interview the senior and family about their values and resources. After reviewing the available living situations in the family and in the desired community, the geriatrics team suggests care sites that keep everyone safe with a lifestyle the senior values.

If your doctor does not have specific training in geriatrics, she should be able to give you a referral to a geriatrics team. If not, you can find geriatrics programs at most university medical centers, through health system physician referral lines, local medical societies, Departments on Aging, and Area Agencies on Aging.

I created the term LOCRx. Your healthcare team may not use the term even though they perform the service. As long as their report includes information that answers the ten LOCRx questions I listed, you will have what you need.

Do You Make Mom Angry or Do You Keep Her Safe?

Sometimes, even though the LOCRx recommends a specific care plan, the senior disagrees. It can seem strange or even wrong to give directions to someone who changed your diapers because it seems at odds with the respect and honor our elders are due. One caregiver told me he was uncomfortable insisting on safety issues with his grandfather. This caregiver had never told any elder what to do; he had been raised to always obey without question. I asked him and I ask you, what would make you more comfortable: *an angry grandfather or a grandfather who hurts himself or someone else?*

Pastor Jimmy Evans also writes about the relationship with elders in his book, *Marriage on the Rock.*(12) Pastor Evans clarifies the Bible's teaching to "Honor thy father and thy mother."(13) He says only *children* are told to obey.(14) Remember your *"big-kid"* ears. You are not a child.

Dad Shouldn't Drive Anymore

Most caregivers find it hard to intervene when a senior can no longer drive safely. For many people, driving equals independence. Most drivers resist any effort to limit this activity at any age.

Over the past year, Mr. Oliver often drove too slowly for the posted speed limit, drifted out of his lane, and misjudged distances. He had several near-accidents on his way to church and to weekly breakfast time with his friends at the Veterans' Hall.

Even though Mr. Oliver insisted that these incidents "could have happened to anybody," his doctor ordered a driving assessment that confirmed several problems. Severe arthritis made it hard for Mr. Oliver to turn his neck. Extra mirrors failed to solve the problem because he also had vision challenges: macular degeneration, decreased depth perception, and inability to judge distance. His reflexes were slow and this caused a dangerous increase in his reaction time. He simply could not drive safely.

Mr. Oliver's family consulted a social service agency to arrange other means of transportation. The agency recommended ride-share programs and a combination of family and community resources so Mr. Oliver would not be house-bound. The doctor and family assured Mr. Oliver that he had put in enough time driving everybody else around; it was his turn to have chauffeurs.

When Mr. Oliver still would not agree, the doctor prepared the paperwork to revoke his driver's license. Mr. Oliver still drove his car. His wife took the keys, but he had several other sets. Finally, Mr. Oliver's wife and children met with him to say they planned to disable the car for his safety. The family also contacted the local mechanics so no one would assist him in getting the car repaired. Mrs. Oliver watched their finances and credit report in case her husband tried to buy a new car. Although Mr. Oliver was angry and felt betrayed, he and other motorists were safe.

Mr. Oliver was so angry that he refused to go out. Finally, his remaining Army buddies descended on his house to read him the riot act about feeling sorry for himself. Did he think he was better than his friends? Hadn't Mr. Oliver driven when Bob had knee surgery? Hadn't he pitched in when Mike broke his foot? Why couldn't they do the same for him? Eventually, Mr. Oliver gave in and his friends took turns picking him up for their outings.

****

Some families admit that though they worry about driving safety, they are either afraid to intervene, or don't know how. It is easy to understand why families have trouble curbing a senior's driving activities. Americans have seen independent driving as an inalienable right since Henry Ford made the Model T affordable for the average person in 1908. We have had a love affair with cars ever since. Losing this right can be a life-changing blow to many seniors' egos. It can also represent crippling dependence. For example, some older women have never driven. If her spouse can't drive, the woman is also housebound. No wonder families are reluctant to take the car keys!

Many families say, "It's okay for Dad to drive because Mom is always with him," but why would that offer comfort? Does a sober passenger make a drunk driver any safer? Mom can't make Dad a safe driver unless *she* can stop the car. When families and doctors fail to remove an unsafe driver from the road, people die.

The rates of accidents among older adults has decreased over the past few years. This may be because seniors are more likely than younger adults to take safe-driving precautions like using seatbelts and not driving drunk. Seniors also drive on the highway less often and for shorter distances than younger adults do.[15] Even so, several age-related problems can affect a senior's driving ability. In addition to problems with vision, there may be decreased visuospatial skills: the ability to judge distance, and perceive where an object is in space compared to another object. There may also be joint pain, decreased joint movement, and slower reaction time. Changes in memory, other brain functions, and other medical conditions can decrease alertness and the ability to respond quickly.

Of all drivers, seniors and teenagers have the highest number of driving fatalities. Seniors drive fewer total miles per year than other drivers and though the different types of driving (on highways versus side streets) make comparisons difficult, the data suggest that seniors have more fatalities per mile.[16] Teenagers' driving skills should improve with time and experience. However, when a senior has trouble driving, the physical and cognitive factors (related to brain function) that contribute to the problem usually get worse with time.

The Special Challenge of Drivers with Memory Loss

Many years ago, the news reported several horrible accidents involving older drivers in Chicago during the same week.

****

An elderly gentleman drove down a bike path and killed a jogger. Another senior turned onto a highway off-ramp, killing himself and another motorist. An older woman plowed into a group of people standing at a bus stop, causing several injuries.

More recently, an elderly couple drove around, stopped for gas and snacks, asked for and received directions from several people but were unable to find their way home. After *several days*, they remembered to call family members who had been frantically searching for them. Thank God they were not lost in the winter or in extreme heat.

****

I cringe every time I hear one of these reports because they are avoidable. A driving incident is not usually the first sign of memory loss in a senior. Many families admit that in retrospect, they had seen worrisome changes long before driving safety became an issue. Did Dad start to dress differently? Did he repeat himself? Did Mom stop baking her award-winning pies? Did she mismanage her money?

Even when memory does not seem "that bad," problems with *executive function* can have a serious impact on driving ability. Executive function requires high-level brain activity that involves memory and a complex series of integrated mental steps. The brain takes in new information, filters it through memories stored from past experiences, decides how to react, and selects the resources it needs to respond correctly. Finally, the brain directs the appropriate body parts to react quickly enough to avoid danger. When we drive, all this brain activity must happen in seconds.

We know this kind of judgment and reaction time is beyond the ability of people who are sleepy or under the influence of certain medicines, alcohol, or drugs. [17] Executive function can also worsen in people whose brains have been damaged by depression, dementia, illness, drugs (illegal, over-the-counter, or prescription), stroke, physical or emotional trauma.

There are times when safety requires that we do more than react. We must anticipate. For example, if a ball rolls in front of your car, you stop because you expect that a child might chase the ball into the street. Someone with executive function problems may not stop until she sees the child. Even at twenty miles per hour, this may be too late. Another impaired driver might see the child and not understand how to respond, or he might not be able to coordinate moving his foot from the gas pedal to the brake in time. The result is tragic!

In Chapter Seven: *Alzheimer's Disease and Other Dementias*, you will learn that people with these conditions usually lose executive function and visuospatial abilities before memory and other brain operations. Mom may know who and where she is and still have problems managing her money, cooking, crafting, or *driving* at her previous level of expertise. She may downplay the little fender-benders, or the times she "just got turned around." He may not have told you about them.

If an impaired senior has not yet had accidents, there is no way to predict how the dementia will progress over time. These seniors cannot say, "Watch out! Tomorrow I won't be able to drive safely." We usually find out after the accident when it is too late.

We don't want to impose unnecessary limits on healthy, independent seniors or allow unhealthy seniors to create dangerous situations for themselves or their communities. If there is a concern about driving safety, it is critical to test a senior's driving ability. Leaving an impaired senior on the road operating a several-ton vehicle is as dangerous as leaving him with a loaded gun.

Test Driving Safety

Departments of motor vehicles in many states have policies for testing senior driving. While they test vision and familiarity with road signs and rules, these tests usually fail to examine executive function. This oversight can leave unsafe senior drivers on the road.

The American Medical Association (AMA) developed a program to help doctors assess driving safety. This publication includes information about testing and recommendations for other resources to provide transportation. (See RESOURCES)

Rehabilitation centers offer comprehensive testing for driving safety. Occupational therapists test vision and hearing, brain function, attention, reaction time, and several types of mobility. These programs usually also conduct monitored road tests with a therapist in the car while the senior drives in the community. Medicare and other health insurance programs usually cover these tests.

The primary goal of the program is not to revoke licenses but to ensure driving safety. The occupational therapists can recommend equipment designed to improve a senior's driving ability. For example, extra mirrors may compensate for problems with neck motion.

Senior service organizations and motor clubs also offer driving safety courses that teach defensive driving strategies that avoid potentially dangerous situations. The AARP offers the Driver Safety Program (1-888-227-7669).

If the test results show that a senior is unsafe in a way that will not respond to instructions or modifications, caregivers must be prepared to disable or remove the car. You cannot expect an impaired senior to just agree that she should not drive. The impact on ego and independence is too high. If the impairment is dementia, *his brain is broken*. The organ that would allow him to reason and agree is the organ that doesn't work.

Determined, disabled drivers may not care about canceled auto insurance or revoked licenses. In my experience, they *always* have extra sets of keys. Families should tell friends and mechanics about the situation so no one helps the senior repair his car or offers the use of another car.

Limiting the senior's ability to finance a new car requires specific actions, which I will discuss in Chapter Four: *When Seniors Mismanage or Struggle with Money.*

In my practice, many seniors told me, "When I want to go somewhere, I don't want to have to wait for anybody. I want to go when I want to go." It may be difficult, but relatives can often arrange their schedules to share availability and increase flexibility for the senior. Many other seniors have friends and church members who can carpool. There are also taxis, ride-share companies, and other driving services. Local eldercare organizations can help caregivers find transportation resources though this may involve a fee. The most important goal is to make sure seniors will not have to decrease their physical and social activities while you keep them and the community safe.

Mom Shouldn't Live Alone Anymore

Caregivers can feel overwhelmed when older adults need help yet insist they are independent.

****

Mrs. Lowell had been active all her life. Over a few months, her legs began to swell, and she became short of breath. Her family tried to get her to call the doctor. She refused.

One day Mrs. Lowell didn't answer the doorbell; her daughter let herself in with a key and found her mother sitting on her sofa. Mrs. Lowell was breathing rapidly, and her entire body was swollen. Doctors in the hospital found that Mrs. Lowell had congestive heart failure and pneumonia. She spent several days in intensive care before embarking on a slow recovery with several weeks of tests and treatments. Eventually, she was able to sit up in a chair but could not get to the bathroom without two people to help her.

Mrs. Lowell balked when her doctors advised her to enter a skilled nursing facility for rehabilitation. She also rejected offers to move in with one of her children. Mrs. Lowell insisted on going back into her own home, alone. She also refused to hire in-home help, saying, "I'm not going to pay money to have a stranger in my house."

A mental health team examined Mrs. Lowell and found no evidence of confusion or depression. She was simply unwilling to accept any change in her lifestyle.

Mrs. Lowell and her adult children met with the medical team several times. Everyone except Mrs. Lowell understood that her wishes were unreasonable. Her family expressed their unwillingness to help their mother hurt herself and presented two options they *would* support: Mrs. Lowell could either:

- Move in with her daughter, accept a companion, daytime nursing and physical therapy in the home, and rotating evening and weekend coverage from her other children, or
- Enter the nursing home.

They agreed to support her choice to go home if the doctors decided her condition had improved enough to make that a safe choice. There were no other options. Mrs. Lowell did not have the physical ability to get herself home. She was angry but chose the least restrictive option, her daughter's home.

After three months, although Mrs. Lowell's condition improved, neither the doctor nor the family believed it was safe for her to go home alone. When she argued, the family said they would not support a dangerous situation and presented her with another choice. She could stay with her daughter, go home with hired help, or move into an assisted-living community. A grumbling Mrs. Lowell eventually said, "I need my own place, but I don't see any reason to try to keep up that big house." She moved into assisted-living where she continues to do well.

****

If the senior is of sound mind and capable of making his own arrangements, he has the right to make bad decisions. You don't have to like it, and you don't have to help them. Step aside. Just try to keep the lines of communication open. This way, you can step back in with safer options when the senior is unable to put her thoughts into safe action, if she can no longer understand the effects of her decisions, or if there is an accident or an emergency.

Even if a legal document says the senior is not capable, you cannot hold up the paper and say, "This means you have to get dressed now." You will need to convince him to cooperate.

Communicate for Cooperation, but Why Would They Listen to You?

Today's seniors include members of the Great Generation whose members were deeply affected by Depression in the 1930s. In WW II, they stormed the beaches at Normandy and survived the Holocaust in Germany. They also created the post-World War II economic boom, and shouldered both the Civil Rights and Women's Movements. The leading edge of the Baby Boomers will reach age seventy-five in 2021. The preferences, activism, and work ethic of this generation has had great impact on social, economic, and political changes. Most of these intrepid survivors will not take kindly to feeling powerless. They are used to tackling obstacles, and they will not hesitate to attack just because *you* are the current obstacle! Here are some basic rules...

Pick Your Battles

Unless the seniors' wishes are dangerous to them or someone else, caregivers should honor their wishes. (The LOCRx will help here). Don't fight over things that don't matter. If a senior wants to sleep on the floor, cover her up. If he wants to put hot peppers on pancakes, unless he has an ulcer or another medical reason for avoiding peppers, be happy he's eating. This may be inconvenient or disruptive to your schedule. It may also bruise your sensibilities. Even though these are the people who created you, the people you looked up to and wanted to imitate, they are different now and you have to try to get past this.

You do not have to rearrange every minute of your life but when you can, as much as you can, let the senior have her way. It's not giving up; it's giving in. Give in to the reality that you cannot control everything and doing it his way might not be the end of the world.

Give as Many Choices as Possible

Every option should be equally safe and acceptable. Does she want to wear the green shirt or the blue one? Does he want toast or a bagel? Does she want to do this or that, first? Keep to the schedule of his favorite TV shows, activities, and routines as much as possible. Does she have to bathe now or can it wait until after *Judge Judy*? Give him the choice, within reasonable limits, but...

Don't Give Choices They Can't Have

Don't ask if she wants to go to the adult day center when staying home alone isn't safe, there's no money for hired help, and you can't take more time off from work. Go out to breakfast or to a store; end up at the center and let the staff handle the fallout. The staff can often entice the older adult by recognizing a skill and putting him in a position of "responsibility." Also, you may have to entice them with activities they enjoy. "After you get back from the center, we will… (Pick a favorite activity)."

Even if they need help, older adults may feel threatened by a hired caregiver. A stranger is entering their domain, trying to take over! You may be able to soothe seniors' feelings by saying, "Mrs. Helper is coming today to give me a hand with the housework." Many parents will tolerate things for their children that they will not accept for themselves. Mom might be more willing to let the worker help *you*. "Here is a list of other things I thought she should do for me. What do you think? Do you have any other instructions for her?" You may have to be there the first few times. You might have to give Mrs. Helper a key. Be sure of yourself. Present the schedule with confidence and do not waver. At the same time, be careful to…

Watch Your Tone of Voice

A parent's disability often makes a caregiver forget that parents are not peers.

Although you have had to make hard decisions and implement them over your seniors' objections, there is *no* role reversal. No matter how disabled they become, your parents never become your children; they are *always* your parents. Your tone of voice should be respectful, never abrupt, and never patronizing (don't say "honey," "sweetie," or whine, "Oh, Mom."

****

Even when my mother's dementia was so advanced that she no longer recognized me, if I was impatient and spoke too sharply, she would slap me just as fast as she would have when I was a kid.

****

Even though you *are* being a responsible adult and working for their benefit, your senior may still see you as a disrespectful, challenging child. How would he have responded to that kind of interaction when you were eight years old or a teenager? Is there any wonder that she won't take it from you now? Even if your relationship was always relaxed and your parents did not require you to say, "Yes, sir," or "Yes, ma'am," they can take offense if you talk to them as if they have no rights.

Just as in marriage or any other intimate relationship, in eldercare, what you say is often less important than how you say it. Calm, respectful tones are key. Don't argue or ignore how they feel. Validate those feelings. You might say, "I see that this is frustrating you. I wish it didn't have to be this way."

Sometimes, You Gotta Do What You Gotta Do

When you've decided on a course of action and your parents disagree but are not able to take care of themselves, you might have to say, "Yes, ma'am," and go on to do what you need to do anyway. Agreeing in words may work for hiring people, rearranging the house, and buying things. It will not work for bathing, dressing, and other direct personal care. As I have said, managing your expectations, being flexible, and offering enticements may work better.

Please understand that your senior is not likely to *ever* say, "You know, hiring this worker was really a great idea. I'm so glad you thought of it" nor anything else that would soothe you. Get your LOCRx, and you will know what you need to do. Work with a professional eldercare consultant or another social service advisor, and you'll know how to do it. If you haven't done either of these things, do them and build confidence that what you've decided is the right thing to do.

When you have information and resources, you don't need to argue or plead. You're right. It must be this way. Go on and get it done.

Again, Use Your "Big-Kid" Ears

Remember, in Chapter Two: *Should Dad Move In With Us*, we talked about hearing our parent's comments with "big-kid" ears and not reacting as if we were still children? Hearing like an adult is especially important when our seniors don't want us to do what we *must* do to keep them safe. It's difficult for those of us who want our seniors' approval and want them to think we're good kids. It is especially hard for those of us who *were* good kids: stayed out of trouble, went to school, always listened, would never lie to them, and were obedient.

However, when they want to do something dangerous, we *can't* obey. The doctor says he *shouldn't* drive; she *shouldn't* live alone; they *are* messing up their finances. If you do what they tell you to do and leave them in danger, how is that being a good kid?

✳✳✳✳✳✳✳✳✳✳✳✳✳✳✳✳✳✳✳✳✳✳✳✳✳

My mother was no longer a safe driver. She changed lanes without looking and drove either too fast or too slow for the posted speed limit. Even though she'd had a couple of near misses, she refused to give up her car so I arranged to have it "stolen." I also planned to lie, say I had no idea how it happened, and console Mother about how dangerous it was to live in North Philadelphia. Luckily, before I could give my cousin the keys on the appointed night, a childhood friend convinced Mother that he needed a car to get to work. She agreed to give him the car. That worked but if it hadn't, I would have been totally comfortable lying to my mama. I would have made that car disappear and denied any knowledge of the action. I knew it would be easier for me to live with the lie than to get a horrible call from the police or the emergency room.

✳✳✳✳✳✳✳✳✳✳✳✳✳✳✳✳✳✳✳✳✳✳✳✳✳

It's hard to make the tough decisions in the face of your seniors' objections. Pick your battles and give them choices when it is safe to do so. If seniors are of sound mind, they are fully empowered to make bad decisions. Though you don't have to be their partner, they won't like it, and they will find a way to make you pay for it. I always say that obstetrical nurses hand a newborn to the parents with instructions on how to make the kid nuts. They know where your guilt buttons are and will push every one of them.

This can be uncomfortable, even painful, especially if you've always enjoyed your seniors' approval As we have discussed earlier in this book, *remember, you're all grown up now.* Though you may think you need their approval, you don't. You need to get the job done. Once you have your LOCRx and your social service partners, do your homework and investigate your options, you can be confident and strong. Hear with big-kid (adult) ears; give honor and respect even though you can't always give obedience.

Just keep asking yourself: *What will it be easier for me to live with: that my loved one is angry with me or that I let something bad happen to him?*

CHAPTER 4

When Seniors Mismanage or Struggle With Money: *What if They Need Money from YOU?*

M oney misery can add major stress and family conflict to an already difficult caregiving situation. Take one senior with limited income, mix in caregivers' financial responsibilities (mortgage, car and other loans, childcare, after-school activities, teenage car insurance premiums, college fees), and you have cooked up a crisis. It can be a real challenge to protect your finances as well as your senior's.

Seniors Face Financial Ruin: Fixed Incomes + Rising Costs = Disaster

Many older Americans live on fixed incomes that cannot stretch far enough to meet unexpected expenses. For some, even basic needs go unmet. Inadequate retirement savings, health challenges, outdated job skills, and limited employment opportunities make it unlikely that many seniors can increase their earning power. When caregivers want to help, it takes information and planning to do so without compromising their own financial health.

The Death of a Spouse Can Destabilize a Senior's Finances

A leaking roof, a broken furnace, or car problems can send any budget reeling. A spouse's death is often the last straw. The estate pays funeral and burial costs as well as the deceased spouse's remaining medical bills. These expenses decrease the amount available to support the surviving spouse. Rarely will a widow receive her spouse's full pension or Social Security benefits. Her income drops; the cost of food, medicines, and utilities might drop a bit, but other expenses do not. Property taxes, insurance, heating and cooling costs depend on the size of the house, not the number of occupants. There may be new expenses if she hires workers to handle the home and car maintenance that her husband had performed. She is also likely to have health expenses of her own.

****

Mrs. O'Rourke's husband died after a long and unexpected battle with complications from a broken hip.

The hospital bills began to arrive two weeks after the funeral. Within thirty days, Mrs. O'Rourke received notice from her husband's pension board and Social Security about the new monthly widow's benefits she would receive. It was less than two-thirds of the benefits they had paid while her husband was alive. She also learned that a downturn in the performance of financial markets had decreased the value of her own retirement funds. Mrs. O'Rourke knew she could manage with less. Hadn't she and Mr. Rourke done that as newlyweds?

At the end of the next month, she received a second notice on one of the hospital bills. She put it on her credit card, expecting to pay it with her Social Security check. The check came on the first of the month along with other bills. Mrs. O'Rourke started to juggle payments and just couldn't keep up. Soon, she could send only the minimum amount due to the credit card company, and she was often a few weeks late. Several months later, the new credit card bill demanded a higher minimum payment. When she called to complain, she learned that late payments had increased her eight-percent interest rate to twenty-one percent. The bills, notices, and phone calls kept coming.

Mrs. O'Rourke's friend told her about a loan from the currency exchange that would "tide her over" until her next Social Security check. When it came time to repay that loan, Mrs. O'Rourke learned that she owed 400 percent interest, which left even less money for her monthly bills.

She and her husband had been proud to pay off their mortgage twenty years earlier. They had maintained their property and Mrs. O'Rourke was confident about the value of her home as she applied for a home equity loan. She thought her application would sail through at a great interest rate and she'd have enough money to solve all her financial problems. She did not believe that her recent problems would erase decades of excellent credit. She was wrong.

Mrs. O'Rourk's neighborhood was no longer desirable to new buyers; the house was not worth as much as she had expected and the decreased equity would not cover her financial shortfall for very long. Her current credit rating barely qualified for the highest interest rate and the monthly payments would be a hardship. The banker showed Mrs. O'Rourke that even if she could qualify for a better rate and more affordable payments, it would take thirty years to pay off the loan. Mrs. O'Rourke's life insurance policy was too small to cover her funeral expenses and the loan. Her children would probably have to sell the house. Property values were still dropping, so the sale could still leave a sizeable debt.

Mrs. O'Rourke knew her children had financial challenges of their own. She had intended to leave the house to them, free and clear. Now, she covered her face with her hands and cried, "How did I get myself into this situation? Bob would be ashamed of me."

****

Health Expenses Can Bust the Budget Too

Unless seniors have Medicare *and* another health insurance plan, they are essentially uninsured. (Check www.medicare.gov for annual updates on Medicare costs and benefits).

After a relatively small deductible (the amount you must pay before insurance kicks in), Medicare Part B covers eighty percent of the cost of office visits, tests, and other outpatient treatments; patients must pay the twenty percent co-payment out-of-pocket. When people need to go to the emergency room, the services are considered "outpatient." The twenty percent co-payment applies even if the care site is in a hospital building. Emergency care can cost thousands of dollars even before a person gets into a hospital bed; this co-payment can be well out of reach for many elders.

Medicare Part A pays for inpatient hospital care. After a deductible, it covers the first sixty days completely (without co-payment). For day sixty-one forward, the size of the daily co-payment depends on how long you are in the hospital and whether you have used up your lifetime number of days for catastrophic illness.

Health insurance penalizes hospitals for unnecessary inpatient days. If your condition is not life-threatening, doctors may place you in "observation" instead of inpatient care. Under observation, you will wear hospital gowns, eat hospital food, and receive treatment yet insurance companies classify "observation" as *outpatient* care. This can be confusing because you are *physically* in the hospital and can often share a room with someone whose is listed as an *inpatient*.

Observation care is subject to the twenty percent Medicare Part B co-payment and this can be very expensive. Though recent legislation requires hospitals to inform patients that they are in "observation," in the past, a senior would be in the hospital, under observation, and unaware of the growing out-of-pocket costs.

Observation patients and their families were also under the mistaken impression that Medicare would pay for post-hospital services (like skilled care in a nursing facility). However, Medicare covers these services only after an *inpatient* stay. Despite the notification, many families are not only blindsided by hospital bills but they also scramble to fund nursing home care.

Other Financial Dangers

A senior's money meltdown isn't always due to poor planning or unexpected financial burdens. Lower interest rates on investments, fluctuations in stock values, and employers that borrow against and otherwise fail to adequately fund pension programs have had a negative effect on retirement funds. The federal government insures pension funds but not at 100 percent. These factors leave many seniors with fewer retirement dollars than they expected after giving forty years to a company. Instead, of retiring in comfort, many risk foreclosure and homelessness.

Current seniors (Baby boomers and the WW II generation) valued financial responsibility. For many, that fiscal discipline resulted in home ownership, which became part of their retirement strategy. With fully paid mortgages and excellent credit, these seniors may qualify for home equity loans and credit cards that they use to pay unexpected bills. If the disparity between expenses and income does not change, these loans offer only temporary relief and eventually, just add to the list of bills. Too often, elders are able to make only the minimum payment each month; they continue to accrue interest and only chip away at the debt. Late payments incur huge penalties, ruin credit ratings, and hike interest rates, all of which increases the debt. In desperation, some seniors turn to payday loans and car title loans that charge exorbitant interest rates. These dig seniors into an even deeper debt-hole.

Older adults can also get into trouble because of telephone, snail-mail, or email propositions for attractive services that are supposedly "free." The services may include hearing aids or other devices that claim to improve comfort, mobility, or security. The fine print or fast-talking sales pitches are hard enough to understand without the vision, hearing, or cognitive challenges that many seniors endure. Bills and threats come months after the seniors have enjoyed the service and passed a cancellation period that was buried in initial paperwork.

Other dangers come from scammers who impersonate the Internal Revenue Service, Social Security Administration, and other legitimate government agencies. These criminals threaten huge penalties unless people give them credit card numbers or bank account information. Other predators call with terrifying stories of loved ones in danger who need money. Internet hackers also send links that download malicious viruses then, demand payment to unlock the computer.

When Seniors Have Open Purses

Often, seniors enable and even encourage younger adults to take advantage of them. This can cause financial crises for responsible caregivers.

****

Mrs. Green was a divorcee with two sons, both of whom had earned bachelor's degrees at her expense. Over the years, the sons repeatedly bounced back into her home to live "until they got on their feet." While paying no rent, they ate, watched cable TV, and ran up their mother's phone bill. Every few months, Mrs. Green would come home to find that one or both of her sons had gone, without a word of thanks or even goodbye.

They didn't send birthday, Mother's Day, or Christmas greetings. In fact, she never heard from either of them until the next time they needed to "get themselves together." Mrs. Green always complained but never said, "No."

She retired after forty-two years at the post office. Several years later, she decided that her forty-eight and fifty-year-old "boys" needed $50 every week and went back to work as a part-time cashier in a parking garage.

At age seventy-five, Mrs. Green had a stroke that affected her memory and ability to walk. She could no longer work or live alone. She had given her brother power of attorney for health care and finance (documents that give him permission to handle her affairs). He arranged for her to move into a beautiful and well-respected assisted-living community. Neither of the Green "boys" visited their mother in the hospital or in the facility. They did call when they needed money. Mrs. Green became upset when her brother asked for her personal checkbook. He feared his sister's health would suffer if she continued to worry about her sons' circumstances. He also worried that she might run out of money for her care.

****

It's Harder to Get Kicked in the Backside if You Don't Bend Over

Many older adults complain yet won't admit that their adult children are in their pockets by the seniors' choice. They continue to baby "grown folks," crippling them, and bankrupting themselves. These parents do not understand that the minute they pass away, these "kids" will have to learn how to fend for themselves. In my experience, these parasitic people either get it together or attach themselves to some other indulgent person.

Mature adults can learn to love their adult children without continuing to take responsibility for them. Dr. Jane Adams' book, *When Our Grown Kids Disappoint Us*, is a good resource.[18]

****

Mrs. Green told her brother she feared she would never hear from her "boys" if she "cut them off." She did admit to concern about running out of money and she agreed to move her direct-deposit pension and Social Security funds into a checking account that required her signature and her brother's. Necessities and bill-payments would come out of this secure account. They also set up a new personal checking account and arranged a smaller automatic deposit, which Mrs. Green could spend as she saw fit. When that money was gone, there would not be another deposit until the next month.

Through counseling, Mrs. Green came to accept that her sons had already "cut her off" and she could not buy their love. She has yet to completely close her purse though she is finding it easier to say "no." She and her counselor are exploring why Mrs. Green has always felt the need to buy love, how she can learn to forgive herself for regrets in her past, and begin to move forward with joy. Mrs. Green has also become more involved in social activities in the assisted-living community.

****

It is hard to reason with seniors who still see other adults as children to nurture and rescue, especially if the parents believe they must atone for perceived (or actual) poor parenting. In my experience, it is impossible to appeal to offending younger adults because they benefit from their parent's behavior. Still there are ways to...

Stop the Financial Hemorrhage

When seniors continue to support younger adults, you may be able to preserve their funds and dignity (as Mrs. Green's brother did) by negotiating a limited amount of money to remain under the seniors' control. Caregivers can further decrease their stress by disbursing this money at regular intervals (for example, monthly) rather than risking large sums, or forcing the senior to ask for every dime. Once you secure the funds to cover the senior's expenses, you must not censure or try to supervise the personal spending account. Choose an amount that won't have ill effects (or make you nuts) if the senior just blows it. You can always renegotiate when finances change.

Manage Seniors' Demands on Your Finances

When seniors' financial decisions get them into trouble, caregivers often try to help. Many caregivers bail the seniors out until repeated requests for resources threaten the caregiver's other financial responsibilities.

****

Mrs. Jones loved flea markets and garage sales. Every weekend, she and her friends visited two or three locations where there were "such good bargains." She had never worked outside the home and lived on a small widow's pension. She had three adult children including two daughters. Her son, John, was the youngest, and she considered him her "right hand." Every few months, Mrs. Jones called her son for money to pay utility shut-off notices or cover repairs to her home or car.

John had been married twenty years, and the first of his three children had just headed off to college. He and his wife had a good income and were very careful with their finances. Still, they did not see a way to keep up their household, educate all three children, save for retirement, and continue to answer his mother's unpredictable and often sizeable requests for money.

John and his mother had many heated arguments about her financial priorities. She thought he treated her like a child. While he didn't want to alienate his mom by continuing to argue and didn't want her be without necessities, he worried about meeting the needs of his family.

I recommended that John should take this approach:

- Sit down with his wife and agree on an amount they could afford to commit to his mother every month.

- Choose the number of his mother's bills that corresponded most closely to that amount.

- Choose bills that would cause *him* the most stress if they went unpaid.

- Arrange for those bills to come directly to his home and pay them every month without waiting for his mother to ask for money.

John told his mother he wanted to do more to help her and asked if he could take over the two bills he had chosen (the cell phone to be sure he could always contact her and the electric bill to make sure she always had a working refrigerator and air conditioning in the summer). He told her he wanted to have the bills come directly to him so she wouldn't have to worry about them. To reduce the cost of his mother's cell phone, Mr. Jones convinced her to change carriers so he could add another line to his unlimited family phone package. He also arranged a senior discount payment plan for utilities. These economies allowed him to pick up her water bill as well.

At first, his mother asked for money to cover other expenses. When she did, John offered calm concern and said, "I know you're frustrated about this. I've taken care of the phone, electric, and water bills. That frees up X dollars. How do you plan to use that extra money? Could it pay for Y?"

John learned not to feel guilty when his mother asked for additional funds. He didn't get angry. Nor did he back down. After tiring of hearing their mother brag about the arrangement with their brother, his sisters decided to participate in the plan. One took over Mrs. Jones' heating bill with help from a special discount for seniors and a monthly payment plan. The other sister did not have financial resources so she arranged for members of her church youth group to cut the grass, rake leaves, and shovel snow to save her mother the expense of hiring services.

Mrs. Jones still grumbles sometimes. When she does, John and his sisters give relaxed, respectful, and supportive comments. They give gentle reminders of the extra money available because of the bills they manage, and they let their mother figure it out.

✳✳✳✳✳✳✳✳✳✳✳✳✳✳✳✳✳✳✳✳✳✳✳✳✳✳

When faced with constant requests for financial support, decide what you can do and do it regularly, without fail and without waiting for the senior to ask. Some families contribute to an account to use for emergency expenses or disburse a specific amount at regular intervals (monthly, quarterly). However, I always recommend paying a bill instead of giving cash. I also suggest that families choose bills with the greatest impact on the senior's health and safety. For example, picking up long-term care or other important insurance premiums has greater impact than covering a hair stylist's bill.

If you cannot afford to take on a bill, can you give time and take over some household chores (shopping, laundry, lawncare, housekeeping) and reduce the cost of paid services? If you give time, remember that the same principles apply: decide how much time you can afford to commit, set up a regular schedule, follow through, and hold the line against other requests. These limits might feel uncomfortable at first but stay strong. Planning can protect a caregiver's assets from sudden, unpredictable expenses that can break your budget, as well as theirs. You can do it!

Start the Process With Communication

The number of gray-haired greeters at big-box retail outlets confirms poor financial security in retirement. A senior's pride and family attitudes against discussing sensitive topics can make financial conversations difficult. Even so, caregivers should try to be aware of changes in income, expenses, and any new loans or services.

Today's seniors come from generations that respected self-sufficiency.

Many are not used to asking for help or taking "handouts." They value solving their own problems and may feel ashamed to share their challenges. They often avoid seeking professional help until the debts and interest have piled up and threatening phone calls overwhelm them.

Attorney Mary Baker (who worked with the former Debt Counsel for Seniors, Veterans and the Disabled [DCSD]) said, "You have to reassure them that they didn't get in this situation by themselves." Ms. Baker recommends that families should *anticipate* financial challenges when a senior has an unexpected or prolonged illness or if one member of a couple dies.

You might start a conversation with:

> "I know that (all these medical bills or other expenses) take
> such a big chunk of Daddy's (Social Security, pension, or other
> resources.) That can make money a little tight. He would want
> you to be comfortable. May I help you look over everything so
> you won't have to worry?"

Another approach might be:

> "Some companies try to take advantage of seniors. They know
> you pay your bills and once they invite you to try their products,
> they sneak in big fees and high interest charges to get you in over
> your head. Then, they harass and threaten you. I don't want you
> to go through that. Will you tell me if anyone offers you new
> credit cards, products, or services, even if they seem to be free?"

Your seniors may balk at first so you will need to keep up a gentle campaign to get the information over time.

We all have experience with loved ones (spouses, children, and parents) who won't listen to us but can hear the same information from someone else. Your seniors may feel more comfortable with a financial management professional. Find well-credentialed, experienced professionals through organizations like the Certified Financial Planner Board (www.cfp.net), National Foundation for Credit Counseling (NFCC), (www.nfcc.org), or the National Association of Personal Financial Advisors (NAPFA), www.napfa.org. Investigate thoroughly before you engage any financial services.

Churches, sororities, fraternities, and other community groups can also be strong resources. Talk to the people in charge of programming for your local organizations and recommend financial literacy topics. (It may work better if you offer the name of a certified professional who is willing to participate.) You can also check with your local AARP chapter about sessions on retirement planning, Internet, telephone, and mail safety, job training, interviewing, and debt management specifically geared toward seniors.

The Guardianship Option

It is more difficult to negotiate a senior's ability to use your funds if the senior is mentally impaired. In that case, you may have to petition for guardianship to protect her physical health, safety, and the funds to provide for her care. The details that follow apply to Cook County in the state of Illinois, where I practiced for most of my career. Local Departments on Aging, eldercare social service professionals, and elder law attorneys have specific information on the guardianship process in your location.

Persons seeking guardianship of an impaired adult engage the services of an attorney to submit the petition and represent them in the proceedings. The process can be complicated; I recommend an elder law attorney who has experience with guardianship, rather than a lawyer whose primary expertise is in tax, real estate, or other areas of the law. (Your state bar association can help.)

Civil court presides over guardianship proceedings. In Cook County, the Office of the Public Guardian becomes involved when the vulnerable senior's estate exceeds $25,000. Either way, the process requires a medical professional to complete a form that documents:

- Whether or not the person is able to make sound decisions to ensure health, finances, nutrition, shelter, and personal safety.

- The cause(s) of any disability.

- If the disability is total or partial and if partial, the types of decisions the person *can* make.

- Whether these causes are irreversible, partially reversible, or totally reversible in an estimated time period.

- The recommended level of care and the appropriate care site.

Medical certification does not assign a guardian; it only informs the court whether or not the senior is incapacitated and *needs* a guardian. The legal system completes the process.

Once someone petitions for guardianship and their attorney files the paperwork, the court appoints a *guardian ad litem*. This is another attorney who protects the rights of the person suspected of being disabled and has no responsibility to the petitioner(s) or anyone else. Then, the court attempts to locate all family members, informs them that the process is underway, and invites their participation.

After reviewing the medical certificate and all other documents, and hearing testimony from all involved parties, a judge makes the decision about the need for a guardian, the type of guardianship required, and whom the guardian should be. The situation can be frustrating because the judge can appoint a guardian who is not someone the caregiver or the senior would have chosen.

Once appointed, the guardian makes all healthcare and financial decisions on the disabled person's behalf. They are accountable to the state and must demonstrate that they have spent the senior's funds solely for that person's direct benefit. Guardians may reimburse themselves for personal funds spent on the senior's needs however, the court requires receipts and thorough, timely reports of all expenses. In some cases, guardians of the person (for health care, personal care, place of residence, and safety) and guardians of the estate (assets and finances) may be different people. They may or may not be required to live in the same state. You will need to review the requirements for your state and county.

The right to make decisions about nursing home placement is not part of an initial guardianship decree. This requires a separate court ruling.

An uncontested guardianship can cost several thousand dollars; the cost escalates if the senior or other parties choose to fight the process. Guardianship can also generate nasty family fights. Caregivers must decide whether they would rather avoid the expense and potential conflict or take a risk that the senior will become penniless and/or unsafe.

You May Want to Make Their Home Equity Work for Them but Consider Reverse Mortgages as the Last Resort

Financial planners warn that seniors should consider reverse mortgages *only* when *no* other assets are available to supplement income or pay extraordinary expenses.

These programs make the equity (net financial value) in a home available to finance caregiving, medicines, or other needs while the senior still lives in the house. The applications do not usually require a credit check, and the government does not consider the funds taxable income. Though these programs may be appropriate for some seniors, the benefit depends on the specific circumstances of the applicant. Pull together your own team of advisors (lawyers, financial advisors, and eldercare consultants) *before* you sign.

There are three types of reverse mortgages...

Home Equity Conversion Mortgages (HECM) are the most common form of reverse mortgages. The Department of Housing and Urban Development (HUD) offers this program and the federal government provides the insurance.

Not-for-profit government agencies offer **Single Purpose Reverse Mortgages** to lower income seniors. Each agency decides the purpose for which its funds can be used, which may include repairs and debt consolidation. For-profit lenders offer **Proprietary Reverse Mortgages,** which may require stricter income/credit application requirements.

To qualify for a reverse mortgage, the senior must be at least sixty-two years old. Banks base the amount of available funds, in part, on the age of the youngest person named on the deed. If your parent is eighty-five and you are sixty-two and a co-owner of the home, the bank will calculate the amount based on *your* age. Usually, the younger the owner, the fewer the available dollars. These contracts lock in the assessed value of the home on the date the reverse mortgage closes. Even if the real estate market improves, homeowners cannot use the increased value unless they pay off the loan, interest and fees, and start over.

The HECM requires each new applicant to review the application with a trained counselor before committing to a reverse mortgage. However, in my experience, these counselors' training includes information about reverse mortgages *only*; they do not usually know about other resources that might help pay expenses, including Veteran's Administration (VA) benefits, state, local, private, or faith-based programs available to older adults.

Many reverse mortgage programs allow owners to live in their homes for the rest of their lives (even if the property has no further value). Unfortunately, these programs do not provide for ongoing maintenance. Once the money is gone, your parent might have a roof over his head but without money for repairs, that roof (and the rest of the house) could fall down around him. Also, since the amount of available money is based on the age of the youngest homeowner and younger applicants are eligible for a lower amount of financing, younger seniors run a greater risk of outliving the available cash.

Some television commercials suggest that people who choose reverse mortgages still own their homes. In fact, *the house belongs to the agency that wrote the mortgage contract.* The senior cannot sell the home or transfer the title unless the terms of the loan are fully satisfied. Full payment includes any funds the senior has withdrawn, all interest that has accumulated since the beginning of the loan, and any penalties for paying the loan earlier than outlined in the initial contract.

Television commercials also suggest that you don't have to pay the loan back. Reverse mortgages are not home equity loans; applicants do not have to repay the money *right away*. Payment is due one year after the last person named on the deed either dies or moves to another permanent residence (nursing home or other location).

If the senior expects to pass the house down to future generations, a reverse mortgage will derail that plan unless the heirs can afford to pay off the loan and all fees. Seniors should learn about their rights and responsibilities, understand how interest rates affect the total payment, and investigate *all* other options before they sign.

****

I was selling autographed books at a women's conference, and my booth was next to Mrs. Dawson, a vibrant, sixty-three-year-old who sold handmade jewelry. Even though her prices were more than moderate, women crowded around her table waiting to buy her unique products.

As we chatted between conference sessions, Mrs. Dawson told me she had just lost her husband of forty years. They raised their children in a home that had been in her family for three generations, and she looked forward to handing it down to her granddaughter. She said she no longer received her late husband's full Social Security benefits and planned to manage her expenses through a reverse mortgage.

I told Mrs. Dawson I thought she should investigate other options. As our conversation continued, it was clear that she had not known the average sixty-three-year-old woman has a life expectancy of about twenty years; she could outlive the equity in her home. Neither had Mrs. Dawson understood that at her death, her granddaughter would have a large financial burden if she wanted to keep the house. Mrs. Dawson was not happy with my suggestion that instead of applying for a reverse mortgage, she should speak with a certified financial consultant about whether selling her home might be a better use of its value. However, she conceded that she would not be able to fulfill her dream of leaving the property to future generations either way.

Mrs. Dawson seemed amazed when I told her that the level of her sales suggested she was still in her income-earning years. I thought there was a real chance of turning a well-loved hobby into a strong business. I referred her to SCORE (Service Corps of Retired Executives), an organization that provides courses and consultation about business and marketing plans, as well as two other community programs that focus on entrepreneurship for women. Also, since her husband had been a veteran, I recommended a local eldercare consultant who was expert in VA widow benefits. Mrs. Dawson agreed to contact the business consultants and the eldercare expert to investigate her options.

****

Although many people look to reverse mortgages to ease money woes, financial planners advise people to consider these programs *only* as a *last resort* after they have investigated *all* other options.

Other Threats to Seniors' Property

When seniors need nursing home care, they must use up a portion of their assets before they can qualify for government-sponsored financial assistance programs. This amount is called the "spend-down" and can be a huge portion of the senior's wealth. In most states, this amount includes all assets that have been in the senior's name for at least five years before the nursing home application. Exclusions vary by state and Departments on Aging publish requirements annually. If there is an ancestral home or other generational wealth intended to stay in the family, these assets will be part of the spend-down unless the family has worked with an attorney or estate planner to move the property out of the senior's name prior to the five-year exclusionary period.

****

Mrs. Ellis brought her mother, Mrs. Williams, to my practice because of memory problems; the tests revealed early Alzheimer's disease. Mrs. Williams's parents had left property in Alabama and as the only remaining child, she was the sole heir. I recommended that the family consult a lawyer for powers of attorney and advice about protecting the property through a trust or by transferring the asset into the name of a younger family member prior to the exclusionary period.

I was Mrs. Williams's doctor for eight years; her disease progressed as expected and eventually, Mrs. Ellis could no longer care for her mother at home. Limited financial resources required public aid funding for nursing home care, and Mrs. Ellis was shocked that the procedure involved a lien on the Alabama property. Since the state included all assets the senior had owned in the past five years, it was too late to move the land out of Mrs. William's name.

Although I had reminded her frequently over the years, Mrs. Ellis always procrastinated about seeking legal advice. She said, "I just don't want to take everything away from Mama." Later, Mrs. Ellis admitted that she hadn't wanted to pay the legal fees.

****

When a state includes property in the nursing home financing assessment, it places a lien on the property, which will appear in a title search. If the heirs want to sell even a piece of the property, the proceeds repay the state before the family gets a dime. Even if they never want to sell, if they want to get a loan to maintain or improve the property, banks are unlikely to accept the value of the home as collateral. In the event of a default, the state's claim would take precedence over the bank's right to recoup its funds.

Instead of waiting for financial crisis, disability, or death to limit your options, work to stabilize your seniors' finances, and decrease their dependence on your assets now. If your family has property to pass on to future generations, it is never too early to consult an estate planner about the type of trust or other strategies appropriate to your situation.

CHAPTER 5

Whose Stuff Is This, Anyway? *Take YOUR Issues OUT of Caregiving*

Even though we give care to benefit our seniors, how much of our caregiving feeds our own needs to be helpful, to justify our existence, show that we are worthy, or to revise history? If we don't answer these questions, our needs can conflict with seniors' needs and compromise their care. This increases their suffering and ours.

The Blinding Need to be Needed

For many of us, caregiving is not just about giving good care; some caregivers believe their primary value as a person is in being a helper and fixer. When caregiving is necessary to our sense of self-worth, there can be an unconscious conflict of interest between helping the senior and protecting ourselves. This may blind us to the senior's real needs and make us *less* effective as caregivers.

Gina is a retired nurse who volunteered as an informal eldercare consultant for a woman from her church, Ms. Logan. Though Ms. Logan's heart was strong, she had lung damage from years of smoking. Osteoporosis (thin bones) had caused the collapse of several of the vertebrae (bones in her spine) over time. This caused a deep curve in her back, pinched nerves, severe pain, and weakness in her legs that confined her to a wheelchair. Shoulder arthritis limited the range of motion of her arms; she was barely able to feed herself and needed assistance for all other activities of daily living.

Ms. Logan didn't accept any of that. She approached everything with the same intense self-reliance she had brought to the Air Force in 1941. She refused to admit her disability, and refused to wait for assistance to get up from her bed or wheelchair. She also refused to leave her home for a more supportive environment until she'd had several painful falls.

Gina explored Ms. Logan's Veterans' Administration (VA) benefits and learned that her military pension would not cover twenty-four-hour in-home care. The waiting list for a VA care facility was more than a year-long so Gina located a private assisted-living facility. Ms. Logan's only relative, a nephew, lived across the country. Although he had power of attorney for health care and finance, he had no interest in his aunt other than to tighten the purse strings. His visits were rare and seldom lasted more than a few days.

The relationship between Ms. Logan and Gina deepened into a close, loving interaction, not unlike a mother and daughter. Gina advocated for the senior with healthcare professionals and the assisted-living facility staff. She also dedicated herself to giving Ms. Logan the best possible quality of life (a way of living that one values and believes is worth continuing).

Gina did the senior's laundry, took care of her pets, and purchased necessities out of her own funds to supplement Ms. Logan's limited income. Gina also brought Ms. Logan to her home for holidays. When the transitions proved too difficult, Gina brought holiday meals to the assisted-living facility.

Despite Gina's devotion and visits from a home care physician and a home health agency, Ms. Logan began to boomerang between the hospital and her home. She continued to fall and experienced repeated episodes of weakness in her face and left arm. The weakness did not resolve and eventually, she also had difficulty speaking and swallowing. Even though Ms. Logan said, "I'm getting weaker and weaker, just fading away," Gina disputed her vehement wish to stop "having tests" and going to the hospital. Gina and the home care doctor decided that Ms. Logan should have an MRI "so we'll know what's going on." As the geriatrics consultant, I reviewed the care plan and raised several concerns:

- It was obvious that Ms. Logan was having strokes; confirming this with an MRI would not add to the care plan. With or without the MRI results, it was too dangerous to use blood thinners that might prevent future strokes because her frequent falls increased the risk of injury and serious bleeding.

- The MRI was equally unlikely to provide other useful information.

- Her overall physical condition was so poor that she would not be a candidate for surgery or chemotherapy if the MRI revealed a brain tumor.

- Even if the MRI showed a tumor, Ms. Logan did not complain of headaches or other symptoms of increased pressure on the brain that might improve with radiation, steroid medicines, of other treatments.

- The MRI could cause harm

- An MRI requires a person to lie still for about twenty minutes. Even if she could manage the time, Ms. Logan's arthritis and spine curvature would make the procedure extremely painful.

- Sedation to manage pain could possibly improve positioning but could worsen her lung function. It could also magnify any stroke-related swallowing problems and increase her risk of aspiration pneumonia (inflammation and infection due to getting mouth contents like food and saliva into the lungs).

I determined that the MRI was an unjustifiable burden for Ms. Logan because the risks out-weighed the benefits. I also believed that continuing to return to the hospital could offer no therapy to improve her quality of life. When I recommended hospice (a philosophy of comfort care that can occur in any location), Ms. Logan agreed. Gina resisted and argued against each piece of evidence that further testing and more medicine would not improve Ms. Logan's condition. Gina said, "I have to do something to keep her going. I will not fail to explore every opportunity to help her get better."

I thought Gina also wanted to avoid her own loss and gently opened that discussion. Eventually, Gina said, "What am I going to do? I've been with her every day for all these years." Wiping tears, Gina shared that she had envisioned another career, but her parents insisted on nursing for their only daughter. She said, "From a very early age, I knew they expected me to dedicate my life to taking care of them."

Gina became an accomplished, highly respected nurse, with a brilliant career in clinical practice, education, and administration. She also supported both parents and an older brother through extended illnesses. She chose not to have a family of her own, used all her pension funds for caregiving, and in her seventies, was still working long after her contemporaries had retired.

Except for the financial consequences, Gina never regretted her decisions. "It makes me feel good to know I can help people." Once her family no longer needed her, Gina began to support seniors at her church. That's how she met Ms. Logan.

Once Gina recognized the origins of her need to help, she was able to admit that continuing medical intervention met her need to help more than it served Ms. Logan's interests. She supported the senior's decision for hospice care and Ms. Logan died in quiet comfort in her assisted-living apartment a few weeks later. Gina was at her side.

Gina continues to help other seniors. Armed with clearer insight, she feels more able to avoid future conflicts of interest between her needs and the welfare of her clients.

****

If You Need Them to Soothe YOU

While some caregivers need to be needed, others need to be appreciated or even comforted. This can add stress to the caregiving relationship.

****

Dorothy is an only child who idolized the strong, single mom who raised her. Mom had always been there for Dorothy. Mom worked hard and sacrificed so Dorothy could be comfortable. She advocated for her daughter in school, cheered her, and dried her tears. Now, Dorothy is married, works full-time, and cares for her mother who lives in her own home. Mom has major mobility challenges so Dorothy visits every day, does Mom's laundry, brings groceries, cooks, cleans, and writes out bills. Dorothy also rearranges her schedule to accompany Mom to doctor visits and entertainment venues.

Dorothy loves her mother and is dedicated to caring for her. Still, she finds herself frustrated when Mom resists help with dressing and personal care. This is especially challenging when Dorothy is on a tight time schedule.

"Mom takes so long and I need to get to work on time. Everything would be okay if she would just let me help her."

Dorothy is also ashamed of the anger that erupts when Mom refuses to do the exercises her physical therapist recommended.

"If Mom can't move around and help herself, I won't be able to take care of her anymore. Why doesn't she see that it makes my life harder when she won't exercise? Doesn't she know it would kill me to put her in a nursing home?"

When Dorothy's frustration shows, Mom talks about her friends who did their exercises and died anyway. She also talks about being a burden to her daughter, which upsets Dorothy even more.

"Mom, how can you say that to me! It makes me feel bad. Don't you care how I feel?"

The conversation usually ends in tears for both women.

****

Dorothy is concerned about her mom but sometimes, she is more concerned about herself. She wants her mother to make things okay for her as Mom did when Dorothy was growing up. She doesn't understand that this is not her mother's job anymore. Mom is struggling with her own fears: the loss of her health and mobility, the possibility of having to leave her home, the loss of her friends, and the specter of her own death.

Even though Dorothy's fears and needs are equally important, she needs to admit that her mom is no longer *her* caregiver. Dorothy must explore other options to manage the logistics of caregiving and decrease her stress. These included:

- Teenagers from the church youth group to help with laundry and grocery shopping after school or on weekends

- A few hours of community care program workers to help with housekeeping, cooking, and daily dressing

- An employee-assistance program consultation to look at flex-time on appointment days

Dorothy should also reach out to friends, caregiver support groups, and counselors to work through her feelings.

By focusing *only* on herself, Dorothy missed opportunities to support her mother. She could have acknowledged her mother's grief, listened to Mom's fears, and soothed *her*. If Dorothy felt that she couldn't do this (or did not want to), she could have recruited clergy, social workers, or counselors to help.

Other caregivers try to change history and the dynamic of their relationship with the senior and seek their approval.

When you Need their Approval

In 2005, Joyce Meyer published *Approval Addiction: Overcoming Your Need to Please Everybody.*[19] While the focus is not on eldercare, I found the book especially helpful for caregivers who need their seniors to see them as "good kids." Many aging parents don't or can't give approval (because of illness, behavioral health issues, or personality). Caregivers' disappointment and resentment can cause pain for seniors and themselves.

****

Mrs. Riley had been an emotionally distant, critical, and unsupportive parent. Her arthritis worsened until it was impossible for her to keep up her house or stand long enough to cook a meal. When two of her three adult children suggested she move into an assisted-living community, the youngest son, Frank, decided to move back into the family home to care for her.

Frank had always felt isolated from his brother and sister because he was eight years younger. The two older siblings were also only eighteen months apart in age, and they were especially close. Frank had been close to their father who had died when Frank was twelve years old. Since his siblings had already left for college, Frank grew up alone with his mother and had borne the full brunt of her personality.

Within three months as his mom's caregiver, Frank sat in his sister's living room, crying as he told his siblings, "I cook and clean. I painted and redecorated to make Mom happy. I buy every movie I think she might like to watch and sit home with her almost every night. My girlfriend threatened to break up with me." His head dropped into his hands as he said, "I promised Daddy I'd watch out for Mom. I don't mean to yell at her, but she isn't even grateful. She told me I was an accident, but I'm the baby. Why doesn't she love me? I thought she would be happy that I'm here, but no matter how much I do, it's never enough."

The older siblings convinced Frank that assisted-living was the best option. They share a visiting schedule and each spends about twenty minutes at a time with their mother. Frank went into counseling and married his girlfriend.

****

Frank desperately wanted his mother's approval. Even though he might not have been aware of it, he hoped to earn her approval through caregiving. He might have fantasized about finally getting a smile from his mother but failed to recognize that she could only be the person she had always been.

You Can Get It Right

One of my mentors cared for her mother in a healthy way.

****

MJ was the oldest of eight children, and their mother had been abusive to them all. Mom was a bitter woman who saw only dashed dreams and impossibilities. She always insisted that other people weren't as happy as they looked, either. MJ survived her childhood and tried to mother her siblings as best she could. She moved into a successful career and through counseling, learned to develop strong relationships outside her family. MJ raised her own children and learned to keep healthy boundaries with her mother and the siblings who didn't break free from that influence. She limited contact to phone calls every few weeks and short visits on holidays.

Years of neglecting her health finally caught up with MJ's mom. Emphysema and congestive heart failure made it difficult for her to manage her activities of daily living and kept her housebound. Several of her children tried to stay with her until she wore them out with her demands and angry tirades.

MJ *chose* to reprise her role as the family's "go-to" person. She moved her mother into her home and hired workers to provide personal care and companionship, remind Mom to take medicine, and prepare healthy meals. When Mom was grumpy and demanding, MJ held the line.

"Mom, I don't need to take that from you," she would say in a calm tone. "This is how we're going to do it."

While some of MJ's siblings didn't understand how she could tolerate her mother's thankless attitude, MJ explained, "I don't expect anything else. I know this is who she is."

MJ spent time with her mom *and* continued to maintain safe boundaries: she excelled in fulfilling work, enjoyed her children, grandchildren, and an active social life. She also kept working with her counselor. After several years, her mom went into hospice care. On her deathbed, Mom told MJ, "Thank you. I always knew you'd be the one to take care of me." No one was more shocked than MJ.

****

I want you to take care of yourself, be healthy, rest, and create joy while giving good care. However, healthy caregiving is about balance, which also means you have to realize it's not *always* about you.

In a sense, the seniors have the biggest problem. As hard as it is to take care of them, it's harder to *be* them. After dealing with everything they've lost or will soon lose, most seniors have no energy to deal with your stuff too. They shouldn't have to.

I understand that this is excruciating for caregivers who, as children, were neglected, abandoned, abused, or overly responsible for parents. They may feel that it was *never* about them. The truth is, most of you won't get the deathbed "attagirl" MJ got. These people were not capable of meeting your needs as a child, and if they haven't worked on their issues in counseling, they are not capable of meeting your needs now. They cannot give you closure. You will need to find what MJ found. MJ's strength was acceptance.

Acceptance

I used to think acceptance was settling or giving up until MJ showed me it's giving *in* and understanding that "it is what it is." It's not that "what it is" is okay. It means no matter what you do, the person or situation isn't going to change and that reality doesn't make you a bad person, at fault, or a failure.

Acceptance frees you to move forward. MJ did not try to change her mother. She did not allow herself to be consumed by anger that her mom would not change, or feel guilty because she could not change her mom. Instead, she accepted that her mother *could not* give approval. In counseling, MJ was able to free herself from the stress of needing that approval. She gave good care on her own terms and met her own needs in other healthy ways. You can too.

Counseling can help you learn to accept the situation and move the fear, hurt, grief, and anger to a place where you can heal. You can also find healthy ways to meet your needs. That's how you give good eldercare. When you get help to deal with your frustration, you avoid mistreating your senior. Even if you think they deserve the injury, being judge and jury hurts YOU. Aren't you hurting enough already?

If you cannot find acceptance and get help for your own needs, remember, you do not *have* to assume caregiving responsibility. It might be best for you and your elder that you do *not* take that role. You *will* face legal consequences if you just walk away. Instead, you can call your local Department on Aging and work with them to set up a different care situation.

If you choose to give care, be sure it is healthy caregiving and a not form of the compulsive behavior, codependency.

CHAPTER 6

Codependency In Caregiving.

W hen we link our feelings of worth and well-being to the behavior of another person, we are in danger of codependency.

What is Codependency?

The information in this section comes from the book *Codependents Anonymous* by CoDA$_{(20)}$ and from conversations with John D., to whom I am especially grateful.

The term "codependency" originally described friends and families of people who live with addiction to alcohol or drugs. People in the addict's support system enable the addiction by encouraging self-destructive behaviors or by making it possible for the addict to continue actions that harm themselves or others.$_{(21)}$ These enablers also deny, ignore, excuse, or try to explain away this conduct. Their sense of self-worth and security depends on the addict's needs and they believe they are responsible for the addict's recovery.

The concept no longer applies only to people dealing with substance abuse. Now, it includes any unhealthy relationship in which one person over-functions and moves into the responsibility-space of another person who under-functions. The codependent person may try to control the other or may submit to that person's control. Though some codependents risk their physical safety, this does not always mean physical control. Codependents also tie their mood and value as a person to someone else's needs, behavior, or emotional state. They can drain themselves in more than one unhealthy relationship and stay involved long past the point of their own pain. Codependents will also compromise their financial security to protect others from discomfort and the consequences of inappropriate or destructive behavior.

Codependency can affect many relationships, including romantic unions, platonic friendships, and workplace interactions. Regardless of the type of relationship, codependency leads to unhappy, stressful, unsuccessful, and often dangerous relationships.

Professionals believe codependency begins when children grow up in homes with abuse, addiction, emotional turmoil, indirect or otherwise poor communication, and emotional deprivation. Young children can take emotional responsibility for a parent with an addiction, mental, or emotional illness. Sometimes, these kids take over operational responsibilities too. They get themselves to school, do laundry, cook, shop, and even interact with creditors. They seek to control the chaos around them, avoid the adult's outbursts or discomfort, and perhaps, earn love. These children survive by learning to ignore their need to be nurtured, as well as their feelings of anger, fear, resentment, sadness, and shame. As they grow into adulthood, they continue the familiar coping patterns. While these strategies seem to have protected them from childhood trauma, the underground feelings have been destructive to self-esteem.

Codependency Can Go in Both Directions

Codependent relationships may start when parents indulge minor children, in order to avoid disruptive behaviors, make excuses for that behavior, do homework, complete college or job applications, and intervene in relationships. Remember Mrs. Green from Chapter Four: *When Seniors Mismanage or Struggle with Money*? She is an example of an older adult who is codependent and risks their financial stability to rescue younger adults who "fail to launch" or otherwise avoid adult responsibilities.

It is also easy to see how caregivers can blur the lines between healthy caregiving and codependency, even in situations that do not involve money. All caregivers attend to seniors' needs. However, the situation can slip into codependency when caregivers lose themselves in those needs, accept too much responsibility for the senior's condition, and feel that their self-worth depends on how the senior feels. This is especially dangerous when caregivers imperil their health, finances, jobs, other relationships, and their joy.

Are You Codependent?

People who are codependent are usually unaware that this is the reason for the pain in their relationships. CoDA literature (www.CoDA.org) and Melody Beattie's book, *Codependent No More*[22] offer information that can help you identify whether or not this is a challenge for you. You can also start by asking yourself these questions. Do you:

- Need to be needed?
- Believe people can't make it without you?
- Need to do things for people that they can or should do for themselves?
- Take responsibility and do things that no one has asked you to do and intervene when the problem isn't yours to solve?
- Get angry when people don't follow your instructions or do things *your* way?

Some professionals believe codependency is a type of addiction. Others believe it is at the base of all addiction as codependents seek to numb themselves from the inevitable pain that comes because one person can never control another person's behavior or situation. Look in the RESOURCE section for tools to help you learn more about a journey toward recovery, healthy caregiving, and healthier relationships.

The primary reason for this book is to answer questions caregivers asked about issues that affect them, but I know how uncomfortable many of you feel about focusing on yourselves. The next chapter gives you a break. In this chapter I will answer your questions about a condition that affects so many of the people for whom you give care: Alzheimer's disease and other dementias.

CHAPTER 7

Alzheimer's Disease and Other Dementias

I have found that memory loss generates the most questions and consultation requests from caregivers and seniors. The statistics in this chapter come from the report, Alzheimer's Disease Facts and Figures 2020[23]. The recommendations I offer come from my training and experience from more than thirty years as a geriatrician helping families cope with dementia and as a daughter who navigated my mother's ten-year journey with the disease.

Many professionals and organizations focus on research with the hope that one day, early detection will allow professionals to offer strategies for prevention, as well as effective treatments and perhaps, a cure. I believe that it is critical for seniors and families to participate in research to achieve these goals because dementia strikes fear in the hearts of seniors and their families. It takes a major toll on caregivers, our health system, and the overall economy. It also robs us of the wisdom, experience, insights, and contributions of people who could have had positive impact on the challenges we face in our country and around the world.

Researchers focus on the biochemistry of the brain and how to use that knowledge to combat dementia. While they focus on the "why," in years of clinical practice and family caregiving, I have dedicated myself to the "what now?" My focus is on the behaviors and situations that challenge seniors and their caregivers today.

Reasonable people can agree that both strategies are of critical importance and are undeniably connected. The number of people affected by dementia is rising. This may be due to the growing number of older adults (who are at greatest risk) and to increased awareness that may lead to more diagnoses. We need the information from research and effective caregiving strategies if we are to conquer this condition.

If You Remember Nothing Else, Remember These Four Takeaways

The annual Alzheimer's Facts and Figures reports are thorough and very clear so this chapter will not focus on statistics in great detail. However, I do want to burn four pieces of information into your mind.

1. *Alzheimer's disease and other dementias are NOT normal aging.*
   If humans ever reach the maximum age limit scientists estimate for our species (about 120 years), maybe everyone will develop dementia. This is not true today. While age is the primary risk factor for diseases that affect memory, there is no such thing as "senility." Dementia is related to aging; it is not an unavoidable result of getting older. Despite the terrifying statistics in the Alzheimer's Association report, today, about ten percent of Americans over age sixty-five have dementia. That means about ninety percent do not have dementia. The condition affects about thirty percent of people over age eighty-five, which means about seventy percent in this age group are not affected.

   If a senior develops a sudden change in memory or a new behavior, there is a good chance that dementia is not the cause. It is important to find out because...

2. *People Die of Dementia*
   Despite the research and advertising, none of the current treatments reverse, stop, or change the outcome of dementia. This means that Alzheimer's disease and other dementias are terminal illnesses. The number of deaths from Alzheimer's disease increased 145% between 2000 and 2017; it is the sixth cause of death among adults in our nation and fifth among people over age sixty-five.

3. *If you see something, say something, and do something NOW!*
   If you suspect that an elder has brain problems, move quickly.
   Dementia is not reversible. Though other conditions that affect the
   brain are potentially curable, they can cause permanent damage
   if left untreated over time. Medical professionals help families
   distinguish dementia from reversible conditions so we don't label
   a person with a deadly disease when he could get better. Even
   though there is not a cure yet, early diagnosis allows us to offer
   support, education, and timely care planning. These resources can
   shield seniors and families from physical, financial, and emotional
   hardship.

4. *You are not alone.*
   There are many resources to help you care for your senior and
   yourself. Dementia professionals will perform tests to give you a
   clearer understanding of your loved one's problems. They will offer
   support groups, books, seminars, websites. They will also refer you
   to social service professionals who will guide you as you put the
   most appropriate care plans in place. These experts can direct you
   to organizations that advocate for programs to benefit all families
   that live with dementia. They also know about opportunities to
   participate in cutting-edge research that works toward a cure.

What is Dementia?

The term "dementia" describes a group of diseases that cause decreased
cognition (memory and other brain functions). The symptoms of dementia
are...

ACQUIRED: The diagnosis of dementia assumes that the person
started with normal cognition and the problems are *new*. It can be
difficult to diagnose dementia in people with some forms of congenital or
developmental cognitive disabilities. If the person never had normal brain
function, doctors try to confirm the change with a thorough history of the
person's usual mental ability.

GLOBAL: There are many components to cognition. These include:

- **Level of Alertness**

- **Memory** (short and long-term)

- **Perception** (ability to interpret sensory information). This is not just sight and hearing. It includes **Visuospatial skills** - the ability to see things in three dimensions and understand spatial relationships. Visuospatial skills allow people to safely judge distance and recognize boundaries or edges between spaces and objects. This skill is critical for negotiating stairs, avoiding falls, and improving driving safety.

- **Language**
- **Judgment, reasoning and decision-making**
- **Learning (concepts and tasks)**

Experts usually do not make a formal diagnosis of dementia if the person has only memory loss while all the other areas of cognition are normal. At least two of the other areas of cognition must also be affected.

PERSISTENT: People say that dementia "waxes and wanes." While this is true, and Mom may have good days and bad days, even at her best, her memory and function are *always* worse than when she was healthy. It's not as if she can perform complex mathematical equations one day and doesn't remember the names of her grandchildren the next day.

PROGRESSIVE: The condition *always* gets worse over time. As the condition progresses, Dad's good days are fewer and they are not as good; his bad days get worse and are more frequent.

IRREVERSIBLE: *We do not have a cure, yet.* Dementia does *not* go away. As you read about dementia and go to meetings, you may encounter the term "reversible dementias." This phrase applies to one of the conditions that I call *masqueraders*: illnesses that affect cognition but could be reversible.

The Masqueraders

Delirium

This term applies when conditions outside the brain cause a change in cognition. These include infections, abnormal levels of oxygen, glucose (sugar), minerals, and other chemicals in the blood, side effects of medicines, and other potentially reversible health problems. While *dementia* changes brain function slowly and does not change the level of arousal, in *delirium*, the onset of symptoms is relatively sudden, and the person is often sleepy (or sometimes, extremely agitated).

Delirium complicates recovery from surgery and prolongs hospital stays. Even so, health care professionals often fail to recognize this condition and miss a small window of opportunity to reverse its effects. Prolonged, untreated delirium can have irreversible effects on brain function, especially in people with dementia because their brains are already vulnerable.[24,25,26]

Depression

This illness usually involves deep and prolonged sadness that affects daily living and can lead to suicide. Depression can be difficult to diagnose because the condition may present in different ways in each person. Many people just have vague physical symptoms (body aches, upset stomach, headache, irregular bowel movements) Others report problems with substance abuse, sleep, and appetite (sleeping or eating too little or too much). Some people cannot pay attention, follow directions, or complete their usual activities. People with depression can also have problems remembering, or they can show apathy (no longer care) for activities, values, and even people that used to be important to them. This can lead to difficulties with relationships, work, or managing finances.

Doctors and families should consider depression when sadness is much worse or lasts longer than expected for a specific situation. One example is a prolonged period of grief after a loss. Although there is no way to know how long is too long, no matter how much time has passed, health professionals should consider treating depression (with counseling and/ or medicine) when anyone becomes isolated, endangers his health with self-neglect (eating, hygiene, housekeeping, paying bills, taking medicines, etc.), or talks about suicide. Statistics show that people between age forty-five and sixty-four and people over age seventy-five have the highest rates of suicide[27]. *This group includes caregivers.*

It is easy to mistake depression for dementia because the basic tests require a person to concentrate and follow directions. People who live with depression can perform poorly on these tests because the illness affects those brain functions. Because of apathy, they may not even try.

Minimal Cognitive Impairment (MCI)

Researchers have described a form of brain dysfunction called Minimal Cognitive Impairment (MCI). In this condition, the senior, the family, or close friends may notice minor changes in behavior or function. Though mental status tests may show some abnormalities, the results are not serious enough to support the diagnosis of dementia. Special tests that find early chemical or structural changes associated with Alzheimer's disease are not widely available and are not usually covered by insurance. If a senior is able to take these tests, even if the results are positive, the changes in the person's behavior are not serious enough to cause disability.

Some people with MCI recover; some stay the same, and others progress to Alzheimer's disease. Researchers believe about fifteen percent of people over age sixty-five with MCI go on to develop Alzheimer's disease.

Some people have more severe memory problems than others. This form of MCI is called "amnestic," which researchers associate with a higher risk of progressing to Alzheimer's disease.

Neuropsychological testing is one option to separate the masqueraders from dementia. I will discuss this in the section on how to make the diagnosis.

The Specifics of Alzheimer's Disease

This illness is the sixth most common killer of American adults and the fifth most common cause of death among the over-sixty-five age group. This illness is related to aging and since the baby boom generation includes the largest number of seniors in American history, healthcare advocates expect the number of affected citizens to explode. There are an estimated six million people with Alzheimer's disease in the United States and by just 2050, the number is expected to grow to about fourteen million.

Neurons are brain cells and *neurotransmitters* are proteins that neurons use to talk to each other. *Tau proteins* help maintain the walls of *microtubules,* tiny tubes that neurotransmitters move through as they travel inside the neurons. People with Alzheimer's disease have abnormal tau proteins. Their microtubules collapse and twist into *neurofibrillary tangles* that choke the brain cells from the inside. This interrupts the flow of neurotransmitters and affects cell function.

Dendrites project from the surface of the neurons and are involved in communication between the cells. *Beta amyloid* is an abnormal protein that forms sticky clumps between the neurons in people with Alzheimer's disease. Alzheimer's specialists and researchers call these clumps *dendritic plaques* that also disturb brain function. Although plaques and tangles are markers of Alzheimer's disease, scientists are not certain that these structures cause the disease.

Pathologists are doctors who study body tissues to find evidence of illness and the causes of death. They can see plaques and tangles in brain tissue, but the tests require such a large sample that pathologists can perform the tests only after death. Pathologists have performed autopsies on the brains of healthy older adults, adults with certain genetic conditions, and people with Alzheimer's. While plaques and tangles exist in all brains, with Alzheimer's there seems to be a larger number of these structures, they concentrate in areas of the brain that control high-level brain activities: memory, behavior, judgment, and other complex functions.

Each side of the brain has four lobes: frontal, parietal, temporal, and occipital. The command centers for high-level brain functions are in the frontal and temporal lobes. There are also critical connections through the hippocampus, a structure deep in the brain, near the underside of these lobes. In Alzheimer's disease, the hippocampus is smaller and contains a larger number of plaques and tangles than in healthy brains.

Much of the research on prevention, early detection, and treatment of Alzheimer's disease involves discovering ways to affect the production or action of the abnormal proteins that cause plaques and tangles. Even so, research has not yet given a clear understanding of whether these structures cause the illness, how they affect the process of the disease, or how to prevent or fight it.

Risks of Developing Alzheimer's Disease

Some risk factors for developing Alzheimer's disease are controllable and others are not.

Controllable Risks

Cardiovascular Risks include the conditions that block blood vessels and cause heart attacks and strokes. These include smoking, high blood pressure, high cholesterol, and diabetes. Scientists report that people with these conditions have a risk of Alzheimer's disease above their risk of brain damage due to stroke alone. Some experts even call Alzheimer's disease "type 3 diabetes." Perhaps a sick brain is more vulnerable to the processes that cause plaques, tangles, and therefore, Alzheimer's.

Chronic Traumatic Encephalopathy (CTE) occurs after repeated head injuries that are serious enough to cause concussion (periods of unconsciousness without physical symptoms and signs of brain damage, or abnormal brain imaging tests). Dementia has been diagnosed in professional boxers and football players.[28] Several former NFL football stars showed the same symptoms as people with Alzheimer's disease, and autopsies have demonstrated plaques and tangles in their brains.[29] Researchers around the world study the effects of traumatic brain injury (TBI) in people of all ages. The information suggests that even incidents that seemed minor at the time and occurred years in the past can cause symptoms later.[30]

Uncontrollable Risks

Age

Though the probability of developing Alzheimer's increases with age, the condition is only *age-associated*; it is *not* normal aging. The average age of onset for a typical person with Alzheimer's disease is sixty-nine years, and the disease can progress over twenty years. This is only an estimate because it has been difficult to know exactly when the disease started. The major emphasis in current research is on measuring biomarkers (abnormal proteins in the fluids around the brain, or in brain imaging studies). The goal is to learn to identify preclinical disease (before the symptoms appear).

Gender? Race? Education Level?

Scientists report that Alzheimer's disease is more common in women, people of color, and the less well-educated. Researchers believe the gender statistic is still valid, even after they adjust for the fact that women live longer, and there are more older women than older men.

I believe caregiver issues may falsely increase the number of people diagnosed by gender, race, and education level. Women, people of color, and the financially disadvantaged (who may be so in part because of lower education) are more likely to live alone. [31] One person has a wife or caregiver who says, "Honey, don't wear your flip-flops in the snow. Let's get your boots, and I'll go with you," Another person wanders around in the snow in her flip-flops and the police take her to a hospital where doctors diagnose dementia. The first person goes on to die of other causes without ever being diagnosed while the other person becomes a statistic. I believe social scientists are exploring this question.

Family History

Although people who have a family member with Alzheimer's disease are at higher risk, most people with Alzheimer's disease have no family history. Looking back to identify a family pattern can be difficult because in the past, the health system was unaware of the disease; testing was neither common nor specific. Doctors failed to diagnose many people who had the disease, yet made the diagnosis in some people who didn't have it. As research develops accurate and cost-effective biomarker tests, future doctors will be able to make the diagnosis and find familial patterns more easily.

Genetic Risks

Chromosomes are found inside living cells. Humans have twenty-three pairs of chromosomes; one of each pair comes from each parent. Chromosomes are made up of genes (specific codes) that direct the production of proteins that determine how body systems work.

The risk of Alzheimer's disease is greater in people who have inherited genes that code for beta amyloid and abnormal tau proteins (that cause plaques and tangles). Alleles are different types of the same gene; each allele codes for a difference in the protein. The apolipoprotein E epsilon gene (apoE) codes for tau proteins. It exists in four different alleles some of which code for abnormal types of tau. If you received a copy of apoE4 from both of your parents, you have a much greater risk of developing Alzheimer's disease than if you received a copy from only one parent or if you inherited other combinations of the alleles. Researchers believe genetics account for about ten percent of people who live with Alzheimer's. For these individuals, the symptoms seem to appear at a younger age, and the disease may have a faster, more aggressive course. So far, scientists have identified increased Alzheimer's risk with abnormal genes on several chromosomes. For example, people with Downs Syndrome have three copies of chromosome 21 instead of two, and they have an increased risk of Alzheimer's disease.

Other Types of Dementia

Vascular Dementia

This form of dementia is common in people who have risk factors for heart attacks and strokes. Certain areas of the brain control specific areas of the body. Dedicated vessels bring blood into each area. Blockages in large blood vessels can destroy an area of brain large enough to cause the physical problems most people recognize as a stroke: slurred speech or weakness in the face, a limb, or an entire side of the body.

The large vessels branch off into smaller ones that penetrate deep into the brain. Blockages in these tiny blood vessels cause strokes so small that neither the person nor the caregivers notice. These mini-strokes occur all over the brain rather than in one location so they don't cause weakness in a specific limb. Instead, over many years, thousands of tiny strokes destroy a significant percentage of the entire brain. Even when these little strokes concentrate in a specific area, they tend to cluster deep inside the brain. Here, they interrupt connections that coordinate memory and judgment. This kind of damage causes dementia. Although families are familiar with muscle weakness as a sign of stroke, they don't find vascular dementia as easy to accept.

Although people confuse "mini-stroke" and transient ischemic attack or TIA, they are not the same. TIAs are "threatened" strokes not "little strokes." TIA symptoms typically get better within twenty-four hours, and neither physical examination nor brain imaging tests (MRI [magnetic resonance imaging] or CT [computerized tomography]) show evidence of permanent damage. A stroke causes brain cell death that is permanent and usually is apparent on brain tests.

The MRI is a sensitive test to diagnose strokes yet it may still miss the tiniest ones. These little strokes may cause dementia, even though we can't see them.

Dementia with Fronto-Temporal Degeneration (FTD)

This is a constellation of conditions where deterioration in different areas of the brain cause specific symptoms that can develop before memory loss. Primary Progressive Aphasia (PPA) presents with problems generating and understanding speech. Progressive Supranuclear Palsy (PSP) causes visual disturbances.

People with FTD can also display inappropriate social behaviors (hypersexuality, aggression, or laughter in sad situations) before they develop major problems with memory. The frontal and temporal lobes lose tissue and many of the cells include a specific structure that pathologists called Pick's bodies.

Dementia with Lewy Bodies (DLB)

Another abnormal protein, alpha-synuclein, collects inside brain cells, forming Lewy bodies, which serve as markers for DLB. Lewy bodies concentrate in the cortex (area of the brain that involves complex thinking) and in deeper brain tissues, causing the classic signs of DLB: dementia associated with visual hallucinations and stiff, jerky movements in the limbs and that can look like Parkinson's disease. In fact, it can be difficult to distinguish DLB from dementia associated with Parkinson's disease.

It is important to recognize DLB instead of mistaking it for other forms of dementia, especially if the seniors are easily upset. People with DLB may react badly to some of the medicines doctors usually prescribe to treat agitation, a common symptom in many forms of dementia and other behavioral health conditions.

Dementia with Parkinson's Disease

Alpha-synuclein can also collect in the parts of the brain that make the neurotransmitter, dopamine. This protein is decreased in Parkinson's disease. The lack of dopamine causes jerky, stiff movements, short steps, and a characteristic tremor, described as "pill-rolling."

Normal Pressure Hydrocephalus (NPH)

In this condition, there is decreased absorption of the cerebrospinal fluid (CSF) that circulates around and through the brain and spinal cord. This causes the ventricles (fluid-filled sacks inside the brain) to enlarge and crush brain tissue from the inside. People with NPH show three classic characteristics: dementia, problems walking, and difficulty controlling urine. If doctors diagnose NPH early, a shunt may re-route the fluid, relieve the swelling. and improve the symptoms. Unfortunately, it is often difficult to know when the problem started. By the time symptoms develop, it may be too late for a shunt to have the desired effect.

Creutzfeldt-Jakob Disease (CJD)

CJD is a rare form of dementia in which an abnormal protein called a *prion* makes other proteins unravel. Brain function declines so rapidly that death may occur in a matter of months. Although scientists believe some forms of CJD are genetic, one variant is due to eating animals exposed to a virus that causes mad-cow disease. The electroencephalogram (EEG) often shows a specific pattern that helps in the diagnosis.

Dementia is also seen in people who live with chronic alcohol use, multiple sclerosis, HIV, Parkinson's disease, and other conditions. Even so, the word "Alzheimer's" generates great fear.

"WHEW! The Doctor Said It's Just Dementia; Thank God It Isn't Alzheimer's! NOT QUITE.

Many families express relief that the doctor said "dementia" instead of the dreaded "A" word. They shouldn't. Alzheimer's disease, vascular dementia, FTD, DLB, and the other conditions are all *types* of dementia, just like apples, strawberries, bananas, and oranges are all types of *fruit*. No type of dementia is more or less devastating than the others.

Some families believe other types of dementia will "turn into Alzheimer's." This is not true. Although the types are different, and one will not turn into another, a person may have more than one form of dementia at the same time. This is known as *mixed dementia syndrome*. It may be difficult for doctors to tease out the effect of an individual type.

Except for avoiding the side effects of a common class of anti-agitation medicine in people with DLB and considering a shunt to try to improve NPH, currently, identifying the different types of dementia does not change treatment or outcome. Even though these conditions may start differently, all types of dementia follow a common pathway: they rob people of their independence, pose similar challenges to caregivers, always cause death, and require the same attention to end-of-life concerns.

Testing for Dementia

The newest and most specific testing involves detecting biomarkers (abnormal tau protein and beta amyloid) in the cerebrospinal fluid, which flows around and through the brain and spinal cord. Researchers also use special dyes with advanced brain scans like PET (positron emission technology) and MRI (magnetic resonance imaging) to show increased amounts of beta amyloid, especially in parts of the brain most involved in memory. Unfortunately, these tests are very expensive, and there is limited coverage from Medicare and other insurance programs. Genetic testing is also expensive and not well-covered by insurance. However, with the increase in interest about ancestry, many advertised programs now offer affordable genetic screening for health conditions, including Alzheimer's disease.

Most people work with primary care professionals, geriatricians, or neurologists who order routine blood tests to find potentially curable conditions that could cause delirium. Traditional brain imaging (CT or MRI) helps rule out strokes, NPH, tumors, other abnormal structures, and collections of blood and other fluids that can put pressure on the brain. The professionals also get a clearer picture of elders' brain function over time by taking detailed histories from families about changes in memory, ability to perform daily tasks, and other behaviors.

Neuropsychologists are PhD experts in brain function. Some subspecialize in learning disorders or traumatic brain injury (TBI). Others are expert in dementia. These professionals can distinguish beteen dementia and the masqueraders. However, I believe their ability to determine what people *can* do and *cannot* do makes their input invaluable. When doctors and family caregivers understand the abilities of the person with dementia, care planning improves and stress decreases.

＊＊＊＊＊＊＊＊＊＊＊＊＊＊＊＊＊＊＊＊＊＊＊＊＊＊＊＊＊＊＊

My mother could never remember what she heard, but she remembered what she saw. While there was no point to calling Mother to remind her of something, we could label items and leave lists, calendars, and schedules in strategic locations around the house. When Mother walked into a room, the notes could remind her what she was supposed to do.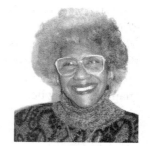

＊＊＊＊＊＊＊＊＊＊＊＊＊＊＊＊＊＊＊＊＊＊＊＊＊＊＊＊＊＊＊

A neuropsychology report can empower families to arrange the senior's environment to play to her strengths (as we did with Mother). This often delays nursing home placement.

Treatment Options

Medicines

Despite advertising for medicines that "treat" Alzheimer's disease, today, no medicine changes the course of the disease; *there is no cure yet.* These "Alzheimer's medicines" (along with medicines that treat anxiety, agitation, and depression) may improve abnormal behaviors and delay a caregiver's decision to use the nursing home.

The most commonly recommended medicines used to cost as much as $280 per month, which in my community would have paid for three or four days of adult day care services. Today the medicine is much less expensive (only about $30 per month). The side effects are not usually dangerous. My greatest concern is that if families believe these medicines cure, they will not see how important it is to plan, hire help, or find other services that support caregivers.

Even if the medicine could make a person with dementia call her caregiver's name 1000 times a day instead of 2000 times, with caregiver support and respite services, the caregiver would not have to hear this at all for several hours or days each week. The caregiver could also use that time to keep her own doctor appointments, go to concerts, play cards with friends, and have a life.

Drug-Free Treatments

Maintaining a well-lit, safe, orderly, and stress-free environment is important in caring for family members with dementia. Keep a regular schedule of meals, activities, and sleep times. Make sure the senior's surroundings have adequate lighting; remove obstacles like toys, junk, loose carpets, and other dangers. Limit irritating stimulation. Noise and crowds are common irritants. Some seniors respond poorly to odors or bright lights and colors. Be mindful of stressors that are unique to your senior. Keep him calm and busy with safe, simple, non-frustrating activities, like folding laundry or snapping string beans.

Phototherapy (Light Therapy)

Circadian rhythm is an internal clock that affects growth in plants and behaviors in animals; it is affected by sunlight. Many people with dementia have a form of circadian rhythm disorder that makes them switch days and nights. This is a major source of sleep disruption for caregivers. I have had some success in resetting internal clocks, using the same kind of light therapy that is effective for treating some people with seasonal affective disorder (SAD-another name for "winter-onset depression"). These people experience depression during times of year when there are fewer hours of sunlight each day (typically, late fall, winter, and early spring). For SAD, some doctors prescribe thirty minutes of phototherapy each morning, using a special box that mimics sunlight without harmful ultraviolet rays. The box should sit about two feet from the person, at eye level without shining light directly into the eyes. (Bulbs for overhead lighting or lamps that shine down onto surfaces don't work. Don't buy them.) Some clinicians (health care professionals who care for patients) believe this therapy improves mood and promotes calmness by changing the levels of the neurotransmitters serotonin and melatonin in the brain. [32] For day-night confusion, I recommend that caregivers schedule thirty minutes of phototherapy in the late afternoon. After a few days, they should try to shift their loved one's bedtime several minutes later and the wake-up time a few minutes earlier every few days until the senior can sleep more continuous nighttime hours.

New medicines for shift-workers and the blind may be of future benefit in adjusting sleep cycles in people with dementia. Unfortunately, the research I reviewed neither includes people with dementia nor considers side effects and interactions with medicines that are common in the elderly.

Before caregivers reach for lights or drugs, they should remember that people are not likely to sleep all night if they nap all day or have a long history as night-shift workers. Caregivers should consider offering shorter, less frequent naps, using adult day services or other activities that keep people awake during the day, or hiring a caregiver who can offer activities at night.

Distraction

Another way to manage agitation is to distract the senior with a new activity or a new subject.

****

My mother did not want to move from Philadelphia to Chicago and she said so, the whole time we packed. Once, when her agitation peaked, I said, "It's cold in Chicago. We already packed your gray coat. You might need another one. Do you want the brown or the red one?" Mother, the fashion plate, said, "Oh, pack the red one, and put this scarf in there too." Every time Mother geared up for a fight, I distracted her with a fashion question, all the way to Chicago.

****

The Most Important Treatment:
Adjusting Caregiver Expectations

Treating the caregiver is often more important than treating the person who has dementia. When seniors no longer function at their best or have abnormal behaviors, many families complain that these seniors are "in denial," "doing it on purpose," "trying to get attention," or "being lazy." This is not the case; *their brains are broken.* Arguing, reminding, harassing, threatening, or yelling never works; if your loved one could remember, learn, or understand, you wouldn't have the problems you have. They can't do it. The connections aren't there anymore.

Even in the earliest stages, dementia has the most devastating impact on the ability to put new facts and situations into memory. People with dementia may be able to recall early life memories until late in the disease because these memories formed before dementia struck. This confuses caregivers who wonder why their loved ones remember things from "back in the day" but cannot remember what happened a few minutes ago. Your dad may always know where he was when he heard President Roosevelt speak about the attack on Pearl Harbor without remembering what he had for breakfast. He may not even remember that he had breakfast.

Although it is hard for caregivers to accept the senior's view of the world, they must learn to do this. Why does it matter if the event happened in 2004 instead of 1947? *You need to go into the senior's reality. You can't bring her into yours.* If the senior says or does something that causes no harm to anyone, let it go.

****

About six years into her ten-year illness, Mother started to put hot sauce on pancakes. She would eat with gusto, without seeming to notice that the pancakes tasted differently. My brother went nuts; I was just happy she was eating and not losing weight.

****

The geriatrics assessment, LOCRx, and neuropsychological testing give caregivers a clearer understanding of what the person with dementia needs and what he *can* do. Learning about the usual characteristics of dementia and the common effects on activity and behavior empowers families to respond to the symptoms more effectively. They can avoid making agitation worse by correcting or arguing. Knowledge tempers expectations and decreases caregiver frustration.

What is "Sundowning?"

Caregivers and other eldercare experts have recognized that confusion and agitation may get worse in the evening. This is called "sundowning" (as it happens when the sun goes down). It can be one of the most frustrating symptoms of all forms of dementia.

Although vision and hearing loss are common among seniors, older adults with dementia may not be able to understand what their senses tell them. When people cannot see clearly, that shadow in the corner may look like a monster, especially in decreasing light (when the sun goes down). If people are unable to hear well, common noises may sound threatening.

Evening is also the time when most family members come home from school and work, yell about homework, share information about the day's activities, bustle around making dinner, and catch up on household chores.

The chaos can further aggravate agitation in a senior with dementia.

Caregivers can address sundowning by making sure there is good lighting and by keeping tabs on their senior's agitation. Mark the times of day when the symptoms seem to be the worst; try to recognize specific triggers and change them as much as you can.

Avoid noise and other provocative factors around the times when agitation is most likely to occur. Of course, you just got home; there are a million things to do, and the work does have to get done. Many older adults enjoy being with their families at this time, but when the commotion troubles the senior, *you* must adjust; people with dementia cannot. Sit her in a separate room, away from the homework, housework, and meal preparation. Try to have someone supervise with a game, a craft, a favorite TV show, music, or another calming activity (like folding laundry). White noise is background sound that does not require direct attention. Many people use static, running water, ocean waves, tinkling bells, chirping birds, and other types of white noise to enhance sleep and improve concentration on studying and other tasks. It may also calm agitation. You can purchase white noise machines from stores that sell electronics.

If you and your doctor choose to use a short-acting anti-agitation medicine, try to give a dose thirty to forty minutes before the senior's most vulnerable time. If you can't pinpoint a vulnerable time, recognize a trigger, or if the treatment plan you develop with your doctor fails, ask whether the side effects of some medicine, a urinary tract infection, or another untreated medical condition could be causing delirium.

The most important thing is to understand that sundowning is common in people with dementia. This might help you control your frustration so you can be more effective in mapping out a strategy.

How Can Someone Die of Dementia?

Remember the four critical points that started this chapter.

1. Alzheimer's disease and other dementias are NOT normal aging.
2. People die of dementia
3. If you see something, say something, and do something NOW!
4. You are not alone.

When families do not understand these four facts, dementia exacts a higher toll on everyone. I have found this to be especially true when people have misinformation about number two. When families are not aware that dementia as a terminal illness, they suffer even more confusion and pain.

****

I was leaving a board meeting when I ran into a friend who had just lost her mother. As I offered my condolences, my friend burst into tears right there in the hallway. Her mother had lived for two years with colon cancer that spread to her liver and bones. My friend said, "Mom's memory had begun to slip even before we found out about the cancer. We thought she was just getting a little forgetful at her age and didn't worry about it." Over the years, though her mother's memory got worse, the family was not concerned until she complained of belly pain. The doctor diagnosed the cancer and the dementia.

Over time, both conditions progressed. Eventually, the doctors told my friend her mother's cancer was stable. They could not predict when the condition would get worse again but at present, no additional treatment or hospital stays were necessary. Her mother was too weak to go home. My friend did not want her elderly father to drive too far to see his wife every day so she moved her mom to a nursing facility closer to the home the couple had shared for sixty years.

Throughout her life, my friend's mother had always said she would want only comfort care if she developed an incurable illness. Weeks before transferring to the nursing home, her mother began to cough when she ate. The condition worsened and respecting the senior's wishes, the family did not place a feeding tube. In less than two months, she died from aspiration pneumonia (inflammation caused by saliva and food getting into the lungs). Guilt compounded my friend's grief because she believed the move had caused her mother's death.

"The doctor said the cancer didn't kill her," my friend said as she cried outside the boardroom. "I was prepared for her to die of cancer, but how can someone die of dementia?"

****

Dementia starts as a cognitive problem (memory loss and decreased brain function). The condition ends as a neuromuscular disease (miscommunication between the brain and the muscles). The disease attacks the most complex brain functions first and moves down the line from more to less complicated activities. Although the destruction is steady, the time course is unique in each affected person.

How Do People Die of Dementia?

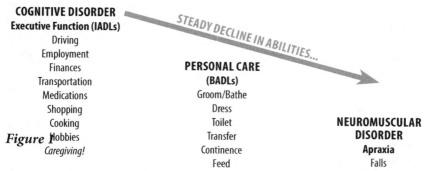

COGNITIVE DISORDER
Executive Function (IADLs)
Driving
Employment
Finances
Transportation
Medications
Shopping
Cooking
Figure 1 Hobbies
Caregiving!

STEADY DECLINE IN ABILITIES...

PERSONAL CARE
(BADLs)
Groom/Bathe
Dress
Toilet
Transfer
Continence
Feed
Aspiration

NEUROMUSCULAR
DISORDER
Apraxia
Falls

Executive function declines first. These are the most complex activities, also called *instrumental activities of daily living* (IADLs). People with intact executive function know what they need to do; they can collect the resources to do it and complete tasks fast enough to avoid accidents or injury. Driving is probably the most familiar IADL. Other examples are: meal-planning, money-management, completing job-related tasks, skills in games of strategy, hobbies, and other recreational activities. People with dementia gradually lose these skills until *basic activities of daily living* (BADLs) begin to erode. These basic skills maintain personal care and decline from the more complex grooming and dressing, to the easiest task of simply putting food into the mouth.(33)

Over time, many people with dementia also face problems with language. In the early stages, though they may have trouble reacting to changes in the conversation and remembering details, they can make common responses, like "Fine, thank you and you?" The ability to use these routine phrases makes their relatives think there is no problem. Healthcare professionals describe this kind of speech as "vacant." As the disease progresses, people may have trouble finding words and often describe the item or its function. For example, if they can't remember the word "pen," they may say, "that thing you write with." People may also substitute words, saying "pen" when they mean "key." Eventually, they may speak nonsense and in the final stages, may become mute. At any stage, people can find it hard to understand language. This leads to major frustration when caregivers believe the senior is ignoring them or "being stubborn."

In the later stages, people develop problems with how the nervous system controls muscles (neuromuscular activity). A normal brain shares information with the rest of the body through continual signals about temperature, discomfort, position, and many other factors that require reactions. For example, a limb tells the brain, "I itch," and the brain sends back a message, "So, scratch," and another limb moves to handle the discomfort. With dementia, the brain either doesn't receive the input, doesn't understand the information, doesn't give effective signals, or the receiving muscle doesn't understand the brain's instructions. Professionals call this *apraxia*. In response to direct testing, the muscles and nerves may work normally but when faced with typical tasks, they don't know what to do. This explains why some people with dementia forget how to use buttons, zippers, toothbrushes, and eating utensils. When apraxia affects the nerves and muscles in the legs, it can cause falls and injuries.

The epiglottis is a muscle in the back of the throat that flips over your airway when you swallow so saliva and food don't get into your lungs. When you breathe, the epiglottis flips over the entrance to your esophagus to keep air out of your stomach. When the epiglottis becomes apraxic (uncoordinated), mouth contents get into the lungs. This is called *aspiration*. Acid in the saliva injures the lungs and bacteria cause infection in the damaged areas. Doctors call this condition "aspiration pneumonia." The infection leaves less space for oxygen and deprives other organs of this life-sustaining gas. *Aspiration pneumonia, is the usual cause of death in dementia.* It is also a complication of strokes and any other condition that decreases the level of alertness. This includes head injuries, abnormal levels of minerals, acids, oxygen, and other necessary substances in the blood. Intoxication with alcohol, other drugs, some medicines, and the effects of certain chemicals can also decrease arousal and increase the risk of aspiration.

****

As I comforted my friend outside that meeting room, I knew her mother's doctors had not helped the family understand that the senior had two terminal illnesses: cancer and dementia. Until I reassured her, my friend thought she had caused her mother's death by moving her to the nursing home. Guilt added to the pain of losing her mother, but this was unnecessary. My friend did not cause her mother's aspiration pneumonia any more than she made the cancer spread. Aspiration was a normal consequence of late-stage dementia.

I also encouraged my friend to value her decision to make things easier for her elderly father. If she had not moved her mother to a closer facility, the daily drive could have proved difficult (and dangerous) for him. Why should she have risked losing them both?

Do I Have Dementia? *A Word of Comfort*

Many people are terrified of developing dementia. This is especially scary for caregivers who watch their parents and other loved ones struggle with the disease. I panic every time I can't find my keys.

Some community health fairs that screen for diabetes and high blood pressure also offer basic memory assessments. I think this is inappropriate because the people who come to these events are not the ones who need it. Even in the early stages of the disease, people with dementia are usually unaware of their problems and see no need for testing. Those who suspect trouble may try to hide their disability and avoid testing. In my experience, the people who present themselves for community-based screening are healthy, worried, and tend to recite long lists of everything they have ever forgotten. These poor folks should take comfort and remember that the primary problem in dementia is memory. *If you remember what you have forgotten, it's probably NOT dementia!*

Though people are afraid of losing memory, luckily most of us have what my Aunt Will called, "Can't remember s_ _t" (I'll call it "CRS.")

How can you tell the difference? I heard Dr. Mladen Golubic from the Cleveland Clinic describe the difference at a conference in 2012. I thought it was so wonderful I decided to borrow it.

CRS   Where are my keys?

MCI   What am I looking for? Oh yeah, my keys.

AD   What's a key?

Even though sudden cognitive changes are more likely due to conditions other than Alzheimer's disease (infections, drug interactions, and other blood imbalances), anyone who worries about signs of dementia should request a medical examination.

How to Get Help

As soon as you suspect changes in a senior's memory or other brain functions, find a team of dementia professionals. Most primary care physicians do not have significant training in dementia investigations. They *can* find illnesses that affect brain function (reversible causes) and offer treatment before these conditions cause permanent brain damage.

If your doctor does not have special training in the care of older adults, is not comfortable diagnosing dementia, or says nothing is wrong when you are still worried, request a referral to a specialist: a geriatrician, geriatric psychiatrist, neuropsychologist, or neurologist. If your doctor refuses and your health insurance requires a referral, contact the health plan for directions on how to appeal that decision.

When your doctor declines your request for a referral and your insurance does not require one, you can find a specialist on your own. Be sure to sign forms that allow close communication between the expert and your primary doctor. This decreases the risk that any part of the care plan will fall through the cracks. It also helps avoid dangerous drug interactions that can occur when one doctor isn't aware of medicine another doctor prescribes.

Don't worry about hurting your doctor's feelings. Your doctor is an adult, and you have the right to advocate for your senior to the best of your ability. Communicate cordially and you will have no reason to apologize for requesting more information.

The Alzheimer's Association can guide you to specialists in your area and is an excellent source for the most current information, resources, and support groups. The Association can also direct you to research centers where you can participate in the latest studies to help find more effective treatments for future families that live with dementia.

Caring for Someone with Dementia - Your Loved One's Brain is Broken

This bears repeating. After a stroke or other brain injuries, swelling decreases and sometimes, other parts of the brain can learn to take over some of the responsibilities of the damaged areas. Unfortunately, with Alzheimer's disease and other dementias, the damage is progressive, and there is no repair. The connections that made your loved one logical, reasonable, or easygoing are no longer working. They won't grow back. Her thoughts, behavior, and function will not improve by reasoning, arguing, or yelling. In fact, loud, emotional interactions can make agitation worse.

As I mentioned earlier, it doesn't matter if the senior with dementia thinks something happened in 1950 when it happened in 1960. *You must go into his reality; he cannot come into yours.* Correcting him just rubs the disability in his face. Older adults will see this as disrespectful, and they can go on the offensive.

My brother in the Spirit, Kirk Riddle, is a Care Warrior who cared for his wife through ten years of Alzheimer's disease. He is one of the most courageous and capable caregivers I have ever known. Kirk recommends that caregivers keep calm and *"Don't poke the bear."* If you know certain things agitate your loved one, try to avoid those circumstances or interactions. If she is already upset, try to remove her from the agitating stimulus: distract her with a new activity, leave the area, stop arguing, and take the conversation in a safer direction.

Even though many of you want to protect your loved one's reputation and legacy you need to protect her physical and financial safety first. *Once you have the diagnosis, do not try to hide it.* Use the third of my Five Keys to Caregiver Survival (See page viii or request a copy of the list at www.drcherylwoodson.com).

3) "Don't Ask; Don't Tell" Won't Work
Tell people you need help.

You need to be open about the condition with people who are in a position to help you make decisions about her future and those who can guide you to the resources you need to give the best care.

****

Lena Hayes was a popular journalist with a syndicated column. She also hosted a national radio show for over forty years. She taught journalism at a local college and mentored several interns at the studio. The radio producers got several complaints about inappropriate remarks, and Lena began to tell off-color jokes on the air. Although her husband thought "those youngsters just want to take her spot," he had to admit that Lena had problems responding to questions from her students and radio callers.

Lena's family arranged a geriatrics assessment that diagnosed Alzheimer's disease. She was not ready to give up her prestigious role, but the college and radio producers were concerned about the complaints. Lena's husband arranged a huge retirement celebration and moved her into emeritus status at the college and radio station. Although she could not cope with the impromptu interactions required to teach or host her show, Lena was still able to communicate her wealth of knowledge about the history of journalism. The family hired graduate students to interview Lena in podcasts and help her organize and edit her written thoughts. She published her column for another year before she retired completely.

****

If seniors with dementia are going to stay on the job, employers, co-workers, and anyone else who interacts with the elder must know the diagnosis and understand the person's deficits.

Full disclosure can result in accommodations that protect the senior's physical and emotional safety while respecting the risk-management policies of the company. It is also important for the senior's financial security. Dementia is a medical issue. Instead of opening pathways to disability and family leave benefits, failure to inform the company about the illness can result in poor performance ratings and disciplinary actions. These can lead to termination and forfeit of important financial benefits (raises, bonuses, and ability to purchase additional life, disability and long-term care insurance).

Remember, you want the company to accommodate, not terminate.

Remember the Four Takeaways

If you take nothing else away from this chapter, remember these four important pieces of information...

1. **Alzheimer's disease and other dementias are NOT normal aging.**
   If a senior develops a sudden change in memory, there is a good chance that dementia is not the cause, but we need to find the cause right away. If the reason is not dementia, we treat. If it is dementia, we plan.

2. **Dementia is a terminal illness.**
   People die of dementia. I have heard many families and doctors say, "He's pleasantly confused." They don't say, "She has pleasantly terminal cancer." It's time to get serious and recognize that changes in brain function are no joke. We need to find answers and get help.

3. **If you see something, say something, and do something NOW!**
   If you aren't sure, find out. You don't want to label a healthy person with a terminal condition. Neither do you want to get help too late to avoid the physical, financial, and emotional hardships that dementia can bring. Get help now. It's better to know than not to know. Don't be afraid to raise calm concern with the family; contact the Alzheimer's Association and other resource organizations to get help. Some of your relatives will bite you at first. They will probably thank you later.

4. **You are not alone.**
   Even if you feel housebound, you can find resources to help you

take care of your senior and yourself. Search the Internet for caregiver chat rooms and webinars. Follow the social media pages and websites of experts in dementia and eldercare. The Alzheimer's Association, AARP, the Caregiver Action Network, and other eldercare organizations have pages on their websites for dementia-caregivers. When you can, attend seminars and support groups in your area (Try libraries and community colleges.) Medical schools with geriatrics programs and Alzheimer's research centers can also offer information and support.

Faith-based communities are stepping up to support family caregivers who struggle with dementia. On the south side of Chicago, several churches from different denominations have banded together to form ta program called REACH - Research and Education for African American Caregivers. This group works with the Mesulam Center for Cognitive Neurology and Alzheimer's Disease at Northwestern University to train volunteers in the health ministries of each congregation to help families recognize dementia and get help. They also co-host a caregiver support seminar series at the Carter G. Woodson Regional Library. The village of Hyde Park has developed faith-based caregiver support coalitions with the Alzheimer's Center at Rush University. You don't have to be a member of a specific church; anyone can reach out and step into a cascade of support, information, and referrals. The village of Lincoln Park and other communities have extensive resources for caregiver education and support as well. It doesn't matter what you believe or where you live; many of us will face dementia-care and we all need help. Go get yours.

Care Warrior, Kirk Riddle, cared for a loved one with dementia. He says, "Alzheimer's wants to claim two victims. Don't let it get you too." The spouse of someone with dementia needs especially compassionate support.

CHAPTER 8

Another Kind of Widow: *When Your Spouse Has Dementia*

Alzheimer's disease and other dementias change the dynamics of relationships long before they claim a person's life. Dr. Jonathan LaPook, (geriatrician and chief medical correspondent for CBS) followed Mike and Carol Daly as they battled Alzheimer's disease together for ten years[34]. Theses interviews clearly demonstrate what Alzheimer's disease and other dementias can do to a marriage.

The grief of a spouse is especially difficult. The spouse loses the special glances and touches, jokes that only the couple understands, bonds forged by years of shared trials and triumph, and the intimacy only lovers can share. Adult children and other caregivers could never know about these cherished details and cannot fully understand the loss. Dementia creates a different kind of widow or widower who needs a unique kind of support.

Today, with increasing awareness among health professionals and families, couples can hear the devastating diagnosis of dementia at a younger age. They can endure the disease through a more sexually active phase of marriage and feel the effects on their relationships for a much longer time. Dementia can make intimacy physically, mentally, and emotionally challenging. For the healthy partner, this often adds to an already painful caregiving situation.

In my medical practice, I worked with several families who grappled with painful issues about physical intimacy, emotional intimacy, and the definition of fidelity.

Although my experience has been with heterosexual couples, I believe these challenges can assault anyone in a committed relationship with someone who struggles with dementia. I welcome opportunities to learn how the LGBTQ perspective is different. Take the recommendations that work for your situation and send your comments through my website www.drcherylwoodson.com.

Your Relationship Changes

****

Mr. and Mrs. Howard had been married thirty years when he started putting his car keys in the refrigerator. After a year of increasingly confused and confusing behavior, their doctor referred them to a memory center at a local university hospital. The team diagnosed Alzheimer's disease, and Mrs. Howard settled into caregiving. She took her husband with her to book club meetings, to church, and on all other errands.

The Howards had always had a rich and satisfying sex life until Mr. Howard's sexual demands increased with his confusion. Mrs. Howard began to feel uncomfortable. She did not want to deny her husband sexual intimacy but in so many ways, he wasn't her husband anymore. His touch was different. He didn't remember what pleased her. Mrs. Howard said she felt like she was being raped every time, and she had no idea how to handle her feelings.

****

Mr. and Mrs. Castor were a power couple. They met in college, married, and carried out their master plan. They each worked while the other finished graduate school; they managed their money, climbed professional ladders, raised and educated their children. The new empty nesters looked forward to more time together and planned a romantic weekend at a local resort.

They motored down the road enjoying their favorite music, but when they approached the first toll booth, Mr. Castor noticed that his wife could not count out the coins.

He became more observant in the next few months and noticed other changes. He found that she needed detailed task lists to complete simple household chores. When Mrs. Castor missed an expected promotion, her husband realized she had a serious problem and began to help her with the paperwork she brought home every night.

One evening, Mrs. Castor called her husband frantic that she couldn't find her way home from work. Even though she didn't know where she was, she was able to describe a landmark. Mr. Castor drove out and found her sitting in her car crying. She was only two blocks from home. The doctor gave the Castors unexpected news that she had Alzheimer's disease at only forty-eight years of age.

Over the next ten years, Mr. Castor took excellent care of his wife. They left their dream home and moved hundreds of miles to be closer to family. He went back to school for a second advanced degree and changed careers to have a more flexible work schedule.

The Castors continued a loving sexual relationship until Mrs. Castor began to seem frightened when her husband brought her to orgasm. She no longer understood what was happening. Mr. Castor felt so guilty about upsetting his wife that after a few times, he stopped trying to share sexual intimacy with her.

****

My heart breaks for Mrs. Howard who endured sexual intimacy with someone who was, in truth, a stranger. I also feel compassion for Mr. Castor who felt like he was raping his wife.

Confusion and discomfort around sexual intimacy were evident in a report about a nursing home that filed charges against an elderly man who continued to have sex with his wife in the facility. (35) The doctors believed the woman's dementia was so severe that she was unable to give consent. The article did not describe evidence of physical force. There no way to know whether the woman welcomed her husband's attentions, or felt coerced, confused, or terrified. Neither did the report reveal the outcome of the court case or the impact on the husband who endured accusations of hurting the woman he had loved for decades. He also had to consider that he might *have* hurt her.

When dementia makes physical intimacy impossible, healthy partners may still have needs. Some decide to meet those needs in another relationship. Others do not. Either way, the decision can bring painful consequences.

****

When Mrs. Castor's dementia became so severe that the adult day care center could no longer accommodate her, Mr. Castor moved her to a nursing home. He visited every day.

Mr. Castor was also my patient. In several office visits, though I tried to discuss his intimacy needs, he always poo-pooed the subject. From age forty on, there are fewer men than women in the US [31]. Even so, Mr. Castor did not believe he would be an object of pursuit for single (and married) women. As I predicted, women came out of the woodwork. Stunned by the number of women who vied for his attention, Mr. Castor struggled with his needs. He rubbed his wedding ring and said he didn't know how to handle his feelings. Then, he lived through a faith-crisis as he agonized over feelings of guilt, abandonment, betrayal, isolation and loneliness before making the difficult decision to start dating.

****

Whether you choose to develop another relationship or not, there are ways to decrease the stress of your decision.

If You Choose NOT to Meet Your Intimacy Needs in Another Relationship

Plan to avoid solitary twosomes. Innocent interactions can change into compromising situations in a heartbeat. In my experience, women know how to dodge these sticky situations while men usually don't have a clue. Here's some specific advice for the guys.

Don't let *any* of the church ladies bring a casserole to "help out." Don't do this at all if you can help it. Definitely, don't let *anyone* stake out her territory by bringing anything or "just stopping by" more than once. Avoid giving rides or answering distress calls. If someone needs help with a flat tire, suggest a roadside assistance company. If they say something is stuck in the sink, suggest they call a plumber. You think this sounds cold? No. It's an investment in your sanity. You'd probably feel worse if you had to get yourself out of an awkward situation or deal with guilt because you succumbed to a sudden urge.

This would also be the time for all caregivers to overcome any shyness and inhibitions about self-pleasure. Ask your doctor about sex toys.

If You Choose to Develop Another Relationship

This decision can also be fraught with guilt and pain.

****

Award-winning correspondent Barry Petersen wrote a book called *Jan's Story: A Love Lost to the Long Goodbye of Alzheimer's.* (37) This is a sensitive exploration of his relationship with his wife, the equally talented journalist, Jan Chorlton. The couple noticed subtle changes in her memory and behavior at age forty and at age fifty-five, they received the diagnosis of early-onset Alzheimer's disease. Mr. Petersen says that Alzheimer's "stole and destroyed . . . a love affair that wasn't supposed to end." After many years, he developed another loving relationship. He continued to love and respect his wife, Jan, as he and his partner worked together to care for her until she died in 2013.

****

Remember Mr. Castor whose wife was diagnosed with dementia in her forties and after ten years, needed a nursing home? He fielded uninvited attention from women until he started dating, met, and fell in love with a woman who respected his commitment to his wife. Friends and family who had comforted and helped Mr. Castor became very vocal in rejecting him. He was devastated until his adult daughter said, "Daddy, Mom wouldn't want you to be alone." With his daughter's support, he nurtured the new relationship and continued to love and advocate for his wife as he always had. Several years later, Mrs. Castor died. Mr. Castor hosted a large, loving homegoing service at their church. A year later, he and his partner married.

****

If you develop a new relationship, prepare for negative and often hurtful reactions from people you had relied on for love, support, and assistance. One caregiver cried in my office after her son said, "Dad's still alive and you're out running the streets!" With time, some of them will come around. You *will* develop new circles of understanding and support, but there can be permanent and painful losses.

It's important to be kind to yourself. Your decision to find another relationship is *not* a sign that you never loved or no longer love your spouse. Neither does it mean that you have lost control or developed strange desires. The need for emotional and physical intimacy is natural, normal, and human. Try to think of this challenge as a dialectic, a discussion of seemingly opposite ideas that can both be true at the same time [38] For example, "I want to stay in bed *and* I have to go to work." You and your spouse share a special bond *and* you have new feelings to explore. Both sides of the argument are true, valid, and important as you decide what behavior is best for you.

It is also essential that you are honest with potential new partners. Make sure they (and you) are clear about your feelings, current responsibilities, and any limitations you place on future commitments. Other people must know whether or not they are in line to become your next spouse. Communication is an investment in avoiding disappointment, broken hearts, and accusations of deceit.

Again, I have a special message for my male caregivers. An unexpected child will add extra levels of responsibility, stress, and potential long-term drama to an already difficult situation. If you become involved with a woman of childbearing age, be clear about whether you want more children. Be vigilant and take active, personal responsibility to avoid unwanted pregnancy. One man in my practice had a vasectomy. Of course, *everyone* should use condoms to protect against sexually-transmitted diseases, which I have diagnosed in patients in their seventies!

The grief of a spouse with Alzheimer's disease is unlike any other kind of grief. Early diagnosis has forced many couples to deal with changes when they are celebrating new freedom from child-rearing. The disease can strike just as the couple is ready to intensify social and sexual activity. Not only do caregiving spouses grieve the loss of the relationship, they struggle with how or even whether to meet their needs for intimacy.

Each caregiver must anticipate these feelings, face them directly, and decide whether to live on one side of the situation or the other. The "right" decision is unique to each caregiver, based on conscience, faith, needs, and other relationships.

Once you decide, commit to behaviors that support your choice. Although you can switch sides as your needs and situations change, it is much more painful to straddle the fence. If you allow yourself to fall off without a plan, your grief, stress, and pain will intensify. You can also hurt others through dashed expectations or unplanned pregnancy.

If your spouse has dementia, please understand that you are not alone.

Your needs are natural; they are not unusual and you should find a safe place to talk about them. Though it is probably not a good idea to start your discussions with family and friends (whose initial reactions of disapproval or anger can cause more stress), don't be afraid. Explore your feelings with a trusted professional and follow the path that's right for you.

When the Person with Dementia Forms Another Attachment

Another painful situation occurs when the affected spouse transfers affection from the healthy spouse to another person.

****

Rev. Gladstone was a powerful and popular pastor whose wife had worked at his side for almost sixty years. Both were active in the community and the couple was well respected.

The head of the deacon board came to Mrs. Gladstone to report that the Reverend was "not himself." He seemed confused during board meetings and did not remember policies and procedures that he had put in place. Rev. Gladstone was an accomplished professional speaker who never used notes but started to write out his presentations. At an outdoor high school graduation, the wind blew away his notes, and he seemed to go blank. He confused everyone by finishing the presentation with a sermon he had given several times in the past.

The doctor diagnosed Alzheimer's disease. Mrs. Gladstone took care of her husband for several years and when she became exhausted, selected an assisted-living community designed for people with dementia.

After a few months, Rev. Gladstone no longer recognized his wife. He believed he was married to one of the other residents, and Mrs. Gladstone was furious. She insisted that the administrator transfer "the other woman" out of the facility. Instead, the administrator scheduled a conference so the families could discuss the situation. Mrs. Gladstone refused to participate.

Since this kind of new attachment is common in dementia-care facilities, the administrator asked the activities director to schedule a screening of the film *Away From Her,* [39] which depicts a similar situation. They opened the activity to residents' families and the surrounding community and invited a social worker to moderate a post-film discussion. Mrs. Gladstone refused to attend.

One day, she saw her husband cuddling with his lady friend and began to scream at the couple. The staff led her away and the administrator suggested counseling.

Mrs. Gladstone admitted to her therapist that the Reverend had not always honored his marriage vows. "I always supported him," she said with angry tears. "I always looked the other way. He never embarrassed me in public before. Why do I have to put up with this now?"

****

Former Supreme Court Justice Sandra Day O'Connor's husband developed this kind of relationship in his dementia-care facility. I am sure Justice O'Connor grieved, but she also expressed happiness that her husband had found some enjoyment in life, despite the debilitating illness.[40]

****

It is painful when a spouse forms another attachment in an adult day program or long-term care facility. Even so, this does not mean that the person never loved *you*. Try to think of this as another type of dialectic. You and your spouse have a loving history, *and* she has reached out to someone else because her brain is broken.

This is especially devastating when there has been a history of infidelity. I always tried to reassure these "widows" that even though the situation raised stinging memories, the spouse was no longer there; he was not capable of handling any kind of confrontation or giving closure. Most of these caregivers required counseling to process their current grief as well as the long-standing hurt and anger.

If you find that dementia has moved you into another kind of widowhood, please don't hold the pain inside. I understand that you might be embarrassed and reluctant to discuss the situation. Still, I hope you will speak with your doctor, a counselor, or another trusted, objective, supportive professional who can help you process your way to peace.

Caregivers who do not get support for their stress, health, and life challenges risk having that stress boil over into elder abuse and neglect.

CHAPTER 9

Elder Mistreatment: Abuse and Neglect Another Form of Family Violence

Over the years, newscasts have reported allegations of mistreatment of aging celebrities. In 2011, famous child star and actor, Mickey Rooney, testified about his experience with elder abuse before the Senate Special Committee on Aging. His stepchildren allegedly intimidated and isolated him, withheld necessities, and misused his money. Mr. Rooney said,

"For years, I suffered silently, unable to muster the courage to seek the help I knew I needed." He said he didn't report because he was, "overwhelmed by fear, anger, and disbelief." (41)

Researchers estimate that six to eight percent of the elderly experience some form of abuse. (36) Factors that affect these numbers may include the growing number of seniors, the challenge of prolonged, disabling illnesses (in all adults,) and the changes in the financial fabric of the nation that have sent many adult children back into their parents' homes (for example, debt, unemployment, under-employment, untreated mental illness, substance abuse, and divorce). Even so, the statistics may only scratch the surface of the problem; like other forms of family violence, victims are reluctant to report elder abuse. Shame, fear (of retribution and of being alone), hopelessness, and being unfamiliar with resources all contribute to under-reporting. Many victims also love the abuser and do not want to upset family relationships or get the abuser into trouble.

****

One of my patients asked an Adult Protective Services (APS) worker not to start the investigation on a specific day because "that's his birthday."

****

Even though many seniors experience elder mistreatment and many caregivers commit this crime, neither party may understand what is happening. Researchers have described several types of elder mistreatment, including different categories of abuse and neglect [42]. If we are to protect seniors, everyone in the family, friends, neighbors, church members, healthcare professionals, community workers, and first responders must have a clear understanding of this insidious and dangerous condition.

Types of Elder Mistreatment

Neglect

There are three forms of neglect that exist when a caregiver fails to meet a senior's needs.

Active Endangerment

Occurs when a caregiver intentionally deprives the elder of essential resources.

Passive Neglect

Involves a caregiver who is ignorant of the care needs, unaware of the means to meet those needs, or incapable of giving care because she is overwhelmed, ill, or disabled herself.

Abandonment

Occurs when a caregiver deliberately walks away from caregiving responsibility without making any preparations for the senior's care.

There is a fourth category of neglect that describes a situation in which there is no caregiver.

Self-Neglect

Exists when seniors fail to provide a safe, healthy life for themselves by declining support or refusing to invest in the necessary resources. Although several states have passed self-neglect legislation, this condition is a challenge to investigate and even harder to address when the older adults have intact mental capacity. When these individuals can understand their options and take responsibility for the consequences of their decisions, they have the right to make those decisions whether or not their choices lead to health, comfort, and safety. Unfortunately, many seniors refuse the physical and mental tests that would confirm or contest their mental abilities.

When families and communities persist in offering help, some seniors accept. However, many seniors are isolated. Even when the elders are not estranged from their families, relatives may not have the financial means to confront the capacity question through the legal system. All too often, these situations end in visits to the emergency department and hospitals, nursing home placement, or death.

Abuse

There are several other categories of abuse, which occur when someone intentionally causes harm, or creates a dangerous situation for the senior.

Financial Exploitation

This is the most common form of elder abuse. Caregivers commit financial exploitation when they use an older adult's resources for *anything* other than the elder's care. It is also exploitation when they spend a senior's assets for goods and services that do not benefit the senior *directly*. The senior may *choose* to share resources however, the situation becomes abusive if the elder does not consent, is not capable of consent (because of physical or mental illness), or feels intimidated or coerced.

Financial exploitation is obvious when someone takes a senior's Social Security check to buy drugs. It is blatant when adult children live at home and use amenities without supporting themselves financially or contributing to the household. Financial exploitation may also appear innocent. If a caregiver uses a senior's money to pay for a cause as worthy as her children's school fees, or if he reimburses himself for travel to visit the senior, *both have committed financial exploitation.*

Physical Abuse –It is NOT Just Physical Injury

Assault

Most people recognize hitting, pushing, burning and other forms of assault as abusive. Other types of physical abuse are less obvious. These include:

Isolation

Denying human contact, in person, by mail, via telephone, or other electronic communication.

Restraint

Restricting movement, for example, tying someone to a chair or a bed.

Confinement

Locking someone in a residence, part of a residence, room, or other enclosed space.

Medication Abuse
Intentional over- or underuse of medicine

Be especially mindful of the potential for abuse even if you restrain, confine, or medicate a senior to avoid agitation or injury. Although you may intend to promote safety, these actions become abusive when used for your own convenience. It is also abusive if these actions endanger the senior for example, leaving them without access to food, toileting, shelter, other comforts, or ability to escape if there is a fire or other emergency.

Sexual Abuse
Sexual contact with a person who is
physically or mentally incapable of consent.

Even without physical evidence of force (bruising or other injuries), professionals consider sexual contact as abusive when mental or physical illness makes consent impossible. Despite the lack of known sexual contact, the diagnosis of a sexually- transmitted disease, or in disabled younger adults, pregnancy, are signs of abuse when the person *cannot* consent.

Psychological or Emotional Abuse

*Yelling, belittling, intimidating, creating an offensive
or hostile environment, or making any kind of threat.*

Most people see threats of physical injury as abuse. They may not understand that threatening to withhold necessities or pleasures is also abusive. Some caregivers make these kinds of threats to force the senior into certain behaviors, however, even when the behaviors are in the senior's best interest, these threats are still abusive. If you tell a senior you won't let him see his grandchildren unless he eats or takes medicine, you have committed psychological abuse.

Different forms of abuse can exist at the same time. Most caregivers do not intend to mistreat their elders; they fail to recognize certain behaviors as neglectful or abusive. They are also unaware of circumstances that pose potential risk for abuse.

* *

Mrs. Farmer had two daughters, Vivian and Linda. Vivian had been unemployed for two years. She and her four children (all under the age of ten) lived with Mrs. Farmer. Linda and her two school age children had been struggling in a nearby apartment until she also became unemployed and moved into the family home. Before her financial distress, Linda had helped her mother pay for medicine and household expenses.

Mrs. Farmer had been independent until a stroke affected her memory and paralyzed one leg. Poor circulation, obesity, and arthritis had already affected her mobility and with the stroke, walking became impossible. She sat in a chair all day, her legs began to swell, and she developed skin ulcers that did not heal. In the hospital, despite intravenous antibiotics, doctors had to amputate her infected leg to save her life. The effects of the stroke and weakness from prolonged bed rest had made her stamina and memory so poor she could neither participate in physical therapy nor learn to use a prosthetic leg. The doctors recommended twenty-four-hour care in a nursing home.

Although the daughters didn't want to leave their mother's care to strangers, they were overwhelmed by her care needs. They agreed to look at nursing homes and thought Medicare would cover the cost until the social worker informed them otherwise. They also learned that since neither of them had been their mother's caregiver for at least three years, they would have to sell the house or pay market-value rent. The proceeds would go to the nursing home, along with their mother's Social Security check. They had no money to pay rent and no household income other than their mother's Social Security benefits so, the daughters took their mother home.

One morning, when the daughters tried to lift their mother out of the bathtub, she slipped and everyone fell. Mrs. Farmer broke her hip and arm. One daughter strained her back; the other one broke her wrist. Despite Mrs. Farmer's fall, her injuries, and increased care needs, Vivian and Linda continued to refuse nursing home care. The healthcare team had no choice. They filed a report with Adult Protective Services (APS).

****

Mrs. Farmer's daughters did not see their behavior as elder mistreatment, but that's what it was. Although they did not intend to be malicious, they committed *neglect* by not providing the care Mrs. Farmer's doctors prescribed. The daughters also relied on their mother's home and Social Security income to support themselves and their children. They did not use the senior's resources to provide the nursing home care she needed. This was *financial exploitation*.

Another Disturbing Type of Abuse

In the last five years of my practice, I saw a different type of elder abuse in seniors who did not seem vulnerable because they were neither seriously ill nor mentally challenged. These older adults didn't need or demand care; they found themselves victimized by criminal relatives.

****

Mr. and Mrs. Kerry had a twenty-four-year-old grandson who had several brushes with the law. The Kerrys hoped to help him escape his dangerous acquaintances and offered him a home with them in another state. Within several months, it became clear that the grandson was not under the influence of bad company; he *was* the bad company. Unsavory characters started visiting the house at all hours of the day and night. Eventually, the Kerrys had several full-time "houseguests." When the seniors complained, their grandson said, "stay out of my business, if you know what's good for you." Intimidated and ashamed to confide in friends, other relatives, or the police, the seniors became prisoners in the bedroom and private bath they had intended for their grandson. He allowed them to use the kitchen twice a day and the laundry room weekly. He also imposed a schedule of when and for how long his grandparents could leave the house. He allowed them to go to the grocery store, the bank, or the doctor with him or one of his "friends." Since they were never alone, the Kerrys didn't say anything to anyone.

The couple had managed their finances at the same local bank for thirty years. A teller became suspicious after several different "grandsons" accompanied one or both seniors to withdraw money. The teller contacted APS, and the workers visited. They alerted police that the young adults refused to let them into the Kerrys' home. They also observed a drug sale on the front steps. The police raided the house and arrested everyone on drug and gun charges. Grandson went to jail, and other family members came to town to help the Kerrys move into secure senior housing. They helped the seniors sell their home to replace some of the funds that Grandson and his criminal friends had stolen.

✳✳✳✳✳✳✳✳✳✳✳✳✳✳✳✳✳✳✳✳✳✳✳✳✳✳

I teach families and health professionals to think about elder mistreatment in a medical model. Just as diabetes, smoking, and high cholesterol increase the risk of heart attacks, certain factors raise the risk of elder abuse. Many of these risk factors respond to prevention in the same way that weight loss decreases the risk of heart disease.

Any situation that increases a senior's care needs and/or decreases the caregiver's abilities should send families, communities, and professionals looking for resources that might avoid danger.

Risk for Abuse

Risks in the Senior

A senior with severe physical or mental illness can generate enormous care needs. Healthier seniors with demanding or abusive personalities can overwhelm even the most capable caregiver.

Risks in the caregiver

Substance abuse and physical or mental illness can decrease a caregiver's ability. Other caregiving responsibilities (multiple seniors, dependent younger adults and/or children) can outstrip the effectiveness of even the healthiest caregivers. Challenges on the job, in relationships, and the weight of other commitments (church, board memberships, volunteer work) can crush caregivers too. Isolated caregivers are at risk if they have no family, if their relatives live far away, or if they are estranged from their relatives. Caregivers can be isolated in dangerous neighborhoods or remote, rural locations. Isolation also occurs when the senior, caregiver, or others in the home refuse visits from people who could give support.

Risks in the family

Though elder abuse can occur in any family, it may be more common in families with a history of other forms of family violence (child or spousal abuse).

Longstanding spousal abuse may continue into late life as "domestic violence grown old." As couples age, either a battered spouse becomes the caregiver for the abuser, or a partner ages, becomes disabled, the abusive spouse becomes the caregiver.[43]

Risk of Financial Exploitation

When caregivers are financially dependent on the senior, a conflict of interest arises that may cause financial exploitation.

****

Recall the Farmer family in the previous example. I do not believe the daughters, Vivian and Linda, intended to harm their mother. I don't believe they saw the situation as a conflict of interest. However, if they had agreed to use a nursing home for Mrs. Farmer, they and their children would have been homeless and penniless. Their financial stability was at odds with their mother's care needs. The conflict affected their decision to keep her at home, which led to financial exploitation and neglect (since they were not equipped to care for her.). The decision also caused everyone to suffer injury.

****

Recognize the Risks for Elder Mistreatment

Although most resources for recognition and investigation are written for professionals, take this information and apply it when you are concerned about a senior in family or your community. I hope by learning this material, you will feel more comfortable referring worrisome situations to social service agencies that can take the investigation further.

Elder mistreatment is a form of family violence that usually involves an imbalance between a senior's care needs and the caregiver's resources. This can happen because the senior becomes more disabled and the caregiver assumes more responsibility or because the caregiver becomes physically, mentally, or financially challenged. An additional risk occurs when there is a history of other forms of family violence.

Imbalance Increases the Risk of Elder Mistreatment

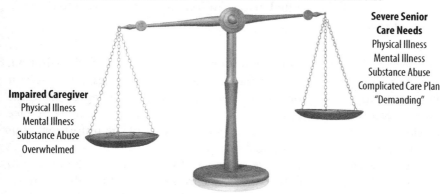

Impaired Caregiver
Physical Illness
Mental Illness
Substance Abuse
Overwhelmed

**Severe Senior
Care Needs**
Physical Illness
Mental Illness
Substance Abuse
Complicated Care Plan
"Demanding"

Recognize Abuse and Neglect

The National Adult Protective Services Association (NAPSA) has comprehensive information about recognizing and reporting elder mistreatment on its website, (www.napsa-now.org).[44] However, other signs may also be of concern.

- Have you not seen the senior in a while?

- In addition to taking note of bruises or other signs of injury, does the senior seems fearful, sleepier, or more confused than usual?

- Take note of *strange or unlikely explanations for a senior's injuries* and be suspicious when the senior, the caregiver, family members, or other witnesses provide different accounts.

- Be suspicious if seniors do not have all their medicines, enough water, healthy, unspoiled, well- prepared food, or the older adult cannot acces the resources. For example, a refrigerator full of food is not useful when the senior cannot walk from the bedroom to the kitchen, her arthritis makes it impossible to open packages, or she has poor cognition and cannot use the stove or microwave.

- Seniors should also have clean, comfortable, weather-appropriate clothing, correct glasses, dentures, and hearing aids, personal hygiene products, and a clean, uncluttered environment with a comfortable temperature.
- Untreated wounds, dirty bandages, poor bowel and bladder hygiene, and untreated health conditions should raise suspicion.
- Professionals should suspect sexual abuse whenever they diagnose a sexually transmitted disease in someone who is too ill to consent to sexual activity.

Several elder mistreatment resources list malnutrition, dehydration, pressure sores, falls, recurrent flares of the same illnesses, and frequent hospital visits as indicators of abuse or neglect. Although I agree that these factors require investigation, I do not think they are *always* definite evidence of elder mistreatment. These findings can be part of the unfortunate but natural course of many chronic diseases.

However, a history of abuse and neglect increases the risk of going to the hospital compared to the risks from chronic illness alone. Research has shown that when social service professionals reported past mistreatment, the senior was twice as likely to suffer future hospital stays than compared to someone of the same age and health conditions who does not have an abuse-report history.[45]

How Do Professionals Investigate Effectively?

Recent changes in health care information systems include elder abuse risk factors questions in patient surveys. Professionals can use many different personal violence assessment tools, however, in my practice, I found these three simple questions most useful.
- Is anyone hurting you or making you feel afraid, uncomfortable, or unsafe?
- Is anyone making you spend money in ways you don't like?
- Does anyone make you do anything you don't want to do or keep you from doing things you want to do?

My medical assistant asked these questions of new patients, of established patients at least yearly, and when any of the staff became suspicious. (Often, the receptionist got the first clue watching the patient interact with the caregiver in the waiting room). I would review the information when I saw my patient. I often heard reassuring statements like, "My daughter won't buy me candy" from several of my diabetic patients. Sometimes, I got information that led to an APS referral.

It is critical for health professionals to *always* interview the senior and caregiver together and separately. This allows observers to see changes in behavior that might suggest abuse. It also gives both parties the freedom to voice concerns they might be reluctant to share in front of the other person. For example, the senior might be relaxed and talkative alone, yet seem fearful or silent in the presence of the caregiver who may also behave differently when interviewed alone. Suspicion should increase if the caregiver is reluctant or refuses to allow separate interviews.

Continual monitoring for caregiver stress can identify risks and allow early intervention to avoid elder abuse and neglect. It is as important to ask the caregiver about her health, stress, and when she last had some fun as it is to ask if the senior feels safe. The American Medical Association (www. ama-assn.org) developed a "Caregiver Self-Assessment" form that I made a routine part of my medical practice. Sometimes, I could get around a caregiver's reluctance about separate interviews by having one of my staff take the patient to another room for a procedure or special test. Then I would say to the caregiver, "This gives me a chance to find out how you're doing. Would you like me to check your blood pressure?"

Report and Treat

Each state has its own laws regarding investigation and intervention. Your local APS program, Area Agency on Aging, or Department on Aging will have information about the reporting requirements and resources in your state.

Anyone in the community can report suspected elder abuse and neglect. Most states require mandatory reporting by attorneys, clergy, coroners, educational system staff, eldercare service providers (licensed or un-licensed), first responders, healthcare professionals, employees, and administrators, social service professionals, and workers in municipal, state, and federal agencies.

Don't Be Afraid to Report

Some people do not report abuse because they don't want to get involved. In most states, potential reporters need not be concerned because the laws allow anonymous reporting and include a "Good Samaritan" clause. This clause protects the reporter from legal charges unless that person would benefit from the report (for example, if the reporter would get control of the senior's finances or other assets).

Other people fear law enforcement problems for the caregiver. However, most states start investigations with a *social service* visit. If a dedicated caregiver lacks information, or there is a stress-related deterioration of a good caregiving system, social service professionals can help families apply for services for the senior. These professionals can also find programs that offer employment, financial, psychological, or substance abuse counseling to stabilize a floundering caregiver. I believe the most effective elder abuse and neglect programs support this social service model with strong law enforcement and legal processes. The combined social service-law enforcement model can encourage reporting by ensuring that caregivers don't go to jail unless that's what they deserve.

****

In the case of Mrs. Farmer and her two daughters, their state followed the social service-first investigation model. Social workers helped the daughters, Vivian and Linda, find income assistance, job programs, affordable childcare, food stamps, and subsidized housing. This released Mrs. Farmer's resources to support the care she needed.

****

Abuse and Neglect in the Nursing Home

Most states handle allegations of abuse in nursing homes through a different process than the one used for community-based reports. For example, the State of Illinois trains and assigns a volunteer ombudsman to investigate these allegations in a specific long-term care site. If the facility refuses to give contact information for the ombudsman or the family is not satisfied with the conversation, the caregiver can contact the Illinois Long-term Care Task Force. Check with your local Department on Aging to learn the rules in your state.

It Takes a Village to Fight Elder Mistreatment

Decreasing the risk of elder mistreatment requires a partnership between caregivers and families, health care, social service, and law enforcement professionals, the community, the legal system, and public policy advocates.

Families and Caregivers

The risk of elder mistreatment increases because of the growing number of seniors, higher care needs associated with chronic illnesses, the ensuing caregiver stress, and caregivers' financial, physical, mental illness. To decrease the risk of elder mistreatment, caregivers should also remember the fifth of my Five Keys to Caregiver Survival (I list all five of the keys on pg. viii or contact me through my website www.drcherylwoodson.com to get your free copy.)

> **5) Put Your Mask on First.**
> (This is what flight attendants tell you to do in case of an emergency).
> *You can't take care of them if you don't take care of you.*

Attend to your own physical and mental health, monitor your stress, and take full advantage of all available support. This decreases the risk of caregiver meltdown that could cause neglect, active endangerment, psychological, or physical abuse. Also, when you take responsibility for your finances, you decrease the risk of committing the crime of financial exploitation.

Professionals

I have found that the weak link in addressing this problem is our system of health care training. We focus on individual hospital stays or episodes of illness instead of looking at the overall pattern. Our system does not always ensure that health professionals follow the same patients over time, and it does not support easy communication between people who give care in the hospital, in the community, in nursing homes, and in other care sites. It is also my experience that the risk factors do not receive much attention in training programs. Though most health care professionals are aware of mandatory reporting laws, many are unaware of the risk factors, the reporting process, and the resources available to intervene.

To avoid the tragedy of elder abuse and neglect, families must have a strong relationship with their senior's healthcare team and feel comfortable asking for help. Professionals should continually monitor risk factors, including caregivers' health and stress-level. As I said before, it is important to interview the senior and caregiver separately as well as together. Both parties may feel more comfortable speaking up and differences in body-language can offer additional information. Ongoing adjustments to the

LOCRx keep families aware of care needs and resources. This teamwork gives professional caregivers many opportunities to assess risk. It also empowers family caregivers to give the proper care, make realistic decisions about whether they can provide it, and explore other options if they cannot.

The Community and Local Governments.

The growing number of mistreatment reports may also reflect the impact of changes in the social fabric of our communities. These include violence, untreated mental illness, poverty, and substance abuse, all of which increase the stress on families. The impact on elder abuse and other forms of family violence due to sheltering-in place from COVID-19 remains to be seen.

Many communities work to address these factors locally while they wait for broader public policy actions from the state and federal government. Interested people should get involved.

I can't overemphasize that it takes the same village to support a vulnerable senior as it does to raise a child. Anyone who comes into contact with seniors should be able to recognize the risk factors for elder mistreatment. If you have any concerns, please contact your local Adult Protective Services (APS) program. Ask for a speaker to come to your church or community organization to raise awareness of the risk factors and resources.

Remember, although laws vary, most states provide for anonymous reporting and protect "good Samaritans." These statutes shield the reporter's identity and protect anyone who files an elder mistreatment report "in good faith," without expecting to benefit. If you have a concern, make the call and make a difference for a senior, for a family.

You *do* make a difference. You pour everything into caring for your loved one and it is often difficult to see a life for yourself outside of caregiving. It is important to develop the other parts of your life so your pain will not intensify when the season of caregiving has passed.

CHAPTER 10

Life After Caregiving:
What Do I Do Now?

Phantom Caregiving and 20/20 Hindsight

Caregivers invest so much of their time, energy, and hearts in caring for loved ones that many feel lost when they no longer have to give care. After all the stress and effort, you would expect caregivers to understand that they deserve to rest. Unfortunately, many don't know what to do with so much extra time when there are no caregiving responsibilities to structure their days. Some find themselves continuing old routines. Others punish themselves by questioning past decisions.

****

Ms. Sawyer was an only child who had always been close to her dad.

"Dad's a pistol," Ms. Sawyer always said. "He regretted not having the confidence to go to college so he never let me back down from anything. Every time I finished something that had that scared me, he would grin and say, 'Easy-peasy.'"

Dad had been a pool shark in his youth. He had never stopped playing for fun and raised his daughter to play well. All through his life, Dad had met his friends at the local pool hall at least twice a week, armed with Delores, his custom-made pool cue.

Ms. Sawyer's father developed Lou Gehrig's disease (ALS, deterioration of nerves in the brain and spinal cord that leads to progressive muscle paralysis and death). His daughter became a strong advocate for him. She kept his health information organized in a ring binder and maintained good relationships with his doctors. Despite her dad's deteriorating mobility, Ms. Sawyer and her boyfriend made sure his life was full for as long as possible: they took him out to restaurants, movies, and plays and often included him in weekend trips to their vacation home on the lake. They also made sure Dad got to see the guys at the pool hall every week. Playing pool became increasingly difficult yet his spirit remained sunny. Whenever he got even close to making a shot, Dad would grin and say, "Easy-peasy."

As the condition progressed, it became difficult for him to perform basic activities of daily living. When even breathing became a challenge for her dad, Ms. Sawyer moved him into hospice care in a nursing facility. She remained an active caregiver and continued the outings until any movement made him uncomfortable.

To the end, Dad never lost his determination or his humor. Whenever someone fed him or helped in any other way, he would flash a bright smile and say, "Easy-peasy."

For several months after Dad died, Ms. Sawyer would get to the grocery store register and see her father's favorite candy in her cart. She would leave work, find herself driving toward the nursing home, and have to change direction. Several times each day, she would pick up the phone to call the nursing home and remember that she no longer had a dad to check on. She also found excuses to avoid spending weekends with her boyfriend at their vacation home. It was too hard to be there without her father.

One evening, as Ms. Sawyer and her boyfriend played pool in their recreation room, she hit a tricky shot, shouted, "Easy-peasy," and collapsed into tears.

"I miss Dad so much," she said as her boyfriend comforted her. "I miss the things we did together. I miss his smile and the funny stuff he'd say, even at the end."

Ms. Sawyer also agonized, thinking she had failed to take some action that would have extended her father's life or made him more comfortable.

"Maybe I should have taken my dad to Mayo Clinic."

"You took the best possible care of your dad," her boyfriend said to reassure her. "The doctors said ALS isn't curable. You couldn't have done anything to change that, Babe, and you did make him happy."

Ms. Sawyer agreed to go to the lake for the weekend, where the couple celebrated her father's life, looked at photos, and laughed about funny "Dad" stories. The next week, she took up her dad's pool cue and began to move beyond her grief.

****

Many caregivers torture themselves with "coulda-woulda-shoulda" and the unnecessary blame adds layers of pain to their grief. Ms. Sawyer might have been able to do something to give her dad a few more weeks, but ALS is unstoppable. Those weeks would not have changed his future. Nor would they have added quality to his life. Even if Ms. Sawyer did miss something in her dad's care plan, she did her best.

The Danger of Not Letting Go

Once life lifts the veil of caregiving, the transition can be traumatic. Some caregivers cannot make the change.

****

Mrs. Evans and her husband own a two-flat building where they live on the second floor with their two teenage sons. Mrs. Evans and her mother were very close. They talked on the phone several times a day, went shopping several times each week, and attended church together every Sunday.

Three years ago, Mrs. Evans' mother developed multiple sclerosis and moved into the first-floor apartment. Although Mrs. Evans had three brothers, she became the primary caregiver.

"I'm going to take care of Mom," Mrs. Evans told everyone. "She's the sister I never had."

Every morning, Mrs. Evans made breakfast for her mother and helped her bathe and dress. She also adjusted her work schedule to sit with her mother until the healthcare worker arrived. In the evening, Mrs. Evans rushed home from work, cooked dinner for her family, and carried food downstairs to share with her mom. They did jigsaw puzzles, watched movies, or she read to her Mom until it was time to help her get ready for bed. Most weekends, Mrs. Evans declined family outings; she even stopped attending church to spend time with her mother. As Mom's disability progressed Mrs. Evans began to stay with her mother until she fell asleep for the night. Mrs. Evans often fell asleep in her mother's apartment.

Mrs. Evans still spends every night in her mother's apartment, away from her husband and kids, even though her mom passed away a year ago.

****

I have worked with several former caregivers who had difficulty moving on. Some developed deep depression that risked other significant relationships, responsibilities, and even their health. If you do not want to withdraw from the world, you *will* need to move on after caregiving. Don't be afraid to get help from behavioral health professionals.

All Cried Out

Many caregivers don't cry when their loved one passes on. That does not mean that they do not grieve. These caregivers often feel extra stress when people wonder why the caregivers don't cry. These well-meaning worriers do not understand; caregivers cry every minute of every caregiving year.

****

My mother was a powerful presence on the planet, and she developed that energy and determination in me. I would not be who I am; I would never have been able to do any of the things I've done if Beatrice Cothran Woodson had not been my mother. Mother was the renegade in her birth family. Unlike other siblings, Mother refused to enlarge my grandmother's nuclear family when she married. She insisted on moving out on her own to form an independent unit with my father and later, my brother and me. Although we remained an active part of the larger family, this boundary did cause a subtle breach with her sisters.

Mother and I were like sisters until I went to college and realized that I wasn't the thumb on her left hand. She had made me her clone in terms of temperament and independence so, I was surprised that she bristled when I pushed back against her continued influence. She was never shy about voicing her opinions and would ratchet up the emotional pressure whenever I decided to go my own way. We were two powerful women and as we struggled to transition from mother and child to mother and adult daughter, our love bonded us in a sometimes, uneasy truce.

My tears began twelve years before my mother died when I realized she was no longer the woman who had raised me. I scheduled the first dementia tests when she started to ask *permission* to interfere in my life.

I made my own clinical diagnosis long before Mother could no longer manage her finances or drive safely. It was two years before a second set of tests confirmed the diagnosis, but my grief started the minute I suspected Mother's condition. I knew dementia was a terminal illness. Visions of her last days flooded my mind long before she developed word-finding problems (calling mountains "the lumpy things"), long before she didn't recognize her favorite singers, long before she didn't recognize *me*.

Dementia took Mother from me in pieces. I cried (inside and out) that first day. I also cried every time I lost another fragment of her, every day for the ten years we lived with the illness, and every one of the eighteen hours I spent holding her while she died. I lifted my head off Mother's chest right after her last breath and had no tears. I was all cried out.

****

Moving Forward Is Not Forgetting: *Forgive Yourself*

Many caregivers resist moving through grief and into the rest of their lives after caregiving because they believe moving forward is forgetting or acting like the person never existed. It's not.

****

My father dropped dead from a heart attack two weeks after I started medical school in 1978; my mother passed in 2003. Even so, my parents are still with me. I feel them on Mother's Day, Father's Day, their birthdays, their anniversary, and other holidays. I can sense Mother looking over my shoulder when I sprinkle paprika over her signature deviled eggs. I know it's her at Thanksgiving when I feel the urge to put a little extra cheese in her famous mac & cheese casserole. I can almost hear her voice, telling me to make sure to match my eye shadow, lipstick, nail color, and accessories so my outfit would look really sharp.

I feel Daddy's presence when I'm baking. He used to brush egg whites over his yeast rolls so they would gleam and give a little crunch as the butter-drenched, soft center melted in your mouth. He also made the flakiest pie crusts. Daddy is with me every Christmas morning too. I remember his eyes twinkling as he passed out presents, puffed fragrant tobacco into smoke-rings, and whistled around the pipe stem he always held in his teeth.

My mother and father are with me whenever I look in the mirror and in the faces of my children and my grandson. My parents' voices come out of my mouth when I comfort or counsel anyone (and of course, when I fuss at my kids).

Sometimes, the memories come with tears; sometimes, I have none. Either way, I miss Mother and Daddy every day and through sweet memories, I still feel their love. To me, those memories more important than tears.

****

I've heard people say, "don't grieve that she's gone; rejoice that she was here." (some people attribute a version of this to Dr. Seuss). Celebrate the time you had with your loved ones. Keep memories alive by sharing scrapbooks, photo albums, mementos, and stories with family and friends. These activities ease fears about forgetting. They also let everyone share the love and help you feel better about moving forward.

Be Kind to Yourself

Forgive yourself. It is not unusual to slip back into old routines. These echoed actions and triggered memories are not lapses. Once seniors pass on, many caregivers find themselves following old routines or starting familiar though now, useless tasks. This is normal. If it starts to disrupt your life and other relationships, contact a counselor.

Accept the decisions you made. No amount of beating yourself will change what happened. No matter what you *might* have done, you made the best decisions you could at the time given the person you were, information you had, and the way the situation presented itself.

Move forward. It will be easier to do this after caregiving if you make time for yourself, your relationships, and your interests while you are still giving care. Even if you don't have a life during caregiving, you can still get through the after-effects. It's never too late to start taking care of yourself. What activities relax you or give you joy? What new activity did you think about trying? Which friends have you not seen or talked to in a while? Reach out. Try something new, and if you can't, contact a counselor.

Grieve in your own way. Don't let others judge your grief by the number of tears you shed, and don't do that to yourself. Grieve the way you need to grieve. Ignore people who wonder why you don't cry. Also forgive yourself for the times when you can't seem to stop crying. If your grief interferes with work, relationships, or life, see a counselor.

When You Feel Relieved

Caregivers who admit to feeling relieved after caregiving often suffer extreme guilt and need special support. I say "admit" because even though people try to deny these feelings, it is normal, natural, and *usual* to feel moments of relief after caregiving. Of course, this does not mean that you wanted your senior dead. Did anyone ask for the illness that needed caregiving? Was this anyone's life plan? Why wouldn't you want the struggle to be over for you, your family, and your loved one? It's okay.

Some caregivers are relieved because they had a difficult relationship with the elder or did not want to be the caregiver. I remind these caregivers that you *did choose* to give care. Instead of calling the Department on Aging and walking away, arranging a nursing home or another alternative, you did not step aside. You decided to give the best care you could despite your feelings. It's okay to feel relieved. *Forgive yourself.*

If you worry that you did not give the best care you could, ask for forgiveness in whatever spiritual context you follow. If that is not an option for you, try to accept that you cannot change the past. Either way, *forgive yourself.*

Some of you are content *because* you did not give the best care. You believe that's what the elder deserved. I ask you to remember that while that senior may have hurt you, caused your anger, and fueled your resentment and revenge, the person can't feel any of that now. Those feelings still affect *you.* By continuing to feed these emotions, you *allow* that person to have continued power over you. You also give them power to affect other people through you. Please work with a counselor to move the pain out of your way so you can go forward into healthier relationships.

Remember, there IS life after caregiving

There must be. So many of us find ourselves on the other side of this experience, and we continue to live. Most of us live well.

Moving forward isn't forgetting or letting go. It's accepting that even though the caregiving is over, the relationship lasts. You honor that relationship and your loved one's life by living *your* life with joy. Forgive yourself as you make time for yourself in caregiving *now.* That will make it easier to move forward into your life after caregiving. When you live with joy, you honor your loved one's life. You also protect yours.

Many caregivers need professionals to help them return from the world of caregiving. Do not avoid the help. Seeking professional counseling is not weakness; it takes courage and strength to seek support and after what you've been through, don't you deserve it?

Tears, grief, and unforgiveness are not the only post-caregiving dangers. If you think there was family drama during the caregiving time, just wait until it's over.

CHAPTER 11

Financial And Emotional Fallout After Caregiving: *This Can Destroy Your Family*

aregiving is stressful; grief is painful. When caregiving is over, the pain can be even worse as you try to manage the details your loved one left behind. Questions about finances, property, and other assets can derail the most stable family relationships. These disagreements can sever bonds that take years to heal, if they heal at all.

Caregiving Can Break Family Bonds

****

Mrs. Clarke had two adult daughters. Jerri, the elder daughter, had a history of financial troubles from which her mother had frequently rescued her. The younger daughter, Eva, had always been frugal and financially independent. When Mrs. Clarke learned she had ovarian cancer, she chose

Eva as Power of Attorney for Health Care and Finance. She also made Eva executrix of her will.

One afternoon, Mrs. Clarke told a friend that she would rather go to the hospital than attend an outing they had planned. The doctors found that the cancer had spread to Mrs. Clarke's liver, brain, and bones. They prescribed pain medicine and explained the possible benefits, risks, and side effects of chemotherapy. Within a few days, Mrs. Clarke said she'd had enough. She signed herself into hospice and passed away at home a few days later.

Even though Eva was devastated, she was committed to following her mother's instructions to sell the house and car and settle all debts and taxes *before* splitting the money with her sister in equal shares. She gave Jerri a few thousand dollars right away and deferred all other distributions until she had settled the estate.

The attorney recommended a real estate agent who found that the village had exempted seniors from several property codes. Mrs. Clarke's estate would have to bring the property into full compliance before sale. Eva hired an inspector to find any other violations and a contractor to complete all required repairs.

Within a few weeks, Jerri became angry and demanded more money. She insisted that Eva was "just sitting on" the funds and was "over there livin' large on Mom's money." Eva tried to explain that she wanted "to let Mom pay her own bills so we don't have to." When Jerri did not relent, Eva also asked, "If I give you all the money and the house needs a new roof, will you be able to come up with half of it?" Although Jerri agreed that she would not, she continued to demand money. She even threatened legal action.

This situation compounded Eva's grief over her mother's death, and she decided to let the attorney handle further communication with her sister. She used her mother's money to pay for the necessary repairs to the house and sold the property. She paid all outstanding debts and taxes before asking the attorney to prepare two checks for half the remaining money. The attorney advised Eva to have Jerri sign a document declining all future legal action or demands of money as a condition of accepting the check. The attorney made the delivery and collected the signed document. Unfortunately, the sisters have not spoken since.

✳✳✳✳✳✳✳✳✳✳✳✳✳✳✳✳✳✳✳✳✳✳✳✳✳✳✳✳✳

Family bonds can shear after a death. Even if the family seemed close, grief, regret, fear, other intense emotions and family dynamics can cause strife without warning.

Mrs. Clarke chose the adult child she trusted to handle her affairs effectively. Although she tried to make it easier by preparing legal documents, this did not protect Eva from her sister's accusations and demands for money. Even though Eva was shocked and hurt, she felt grateful for her mother's directions and for support from professionals.

If you find yourself in this difficult situation, don't lead with your emotions. Work with an attorney, realtor, financial advisor, or other appropriate professionals to stand with you as you comply with your senior's wishes and the local laws. It is possible that your family will come around, in time. Until then, you can take comfort in having honored your senior's trust even as you grieve the situation.

Avoid the Fallout

****

One of my mentors has a sizeable estate and several adult children. As she prepared her estate planning, she knew her eldest would feel slighted if she did not pick him as executor. She also knew that several of the others were more skilled at money management. Guilt and fear paralyzed her until I recommended that she appoint a professional to execute the estate. That way, she wouldn't have to choose between her children, worry about how they would spend her money, or fear the effect possible arguments might have on the family she cherished. The children could fight with the trust officer, not each other. That might make it easier to continue their relationships.

****

The best way to avoid family strife after caregiving is to discuss plans when older adults are still healthy. This can be frightening for seniors and adult children alike. The specter of future caregiving can be equally terrifying for younger adults who have no idea how to prepare to care.

CHAPTER 12

Prepare To Care: *For the Future and for Preparing to Care Again Tomorrow*

Anticipating caregiving can be almost as stressful as giving the care. My coach, Monique Caradine-Kitchens, asked me to launch a blog series on preparing to care because she is an only child. Monique said she was anxious about shouldering future eldercare responsibilities alone. She laughed when I said she was in the best possible situation because she won't have to fight with anyone, but I was only half-teasing. I have worked with so many families in open conflict that sometimes, I think it might be better to do it alone. Still, I understand why it is better to have *effective, cooperative* partners to share the physical, financial, and emotional load.

Preparing to care means having information about possible challenges, learning how the senior would want to manage those challenges, and knowing what resources would be available. Many adult children say they don't want to insult their parents by asking health and financial questions. Others ask and feel frustrated when their parents won't tell them anything.

Though some parents believe their adult children are "getting in my business," or "pushing me into the grave," many seniors don't intend to make their adult children's lives more difficult. They may avoid these conversations or refuse to share information because they fear disability or death and don't want to think about either. Others believe death will come sooner if they talk about the possibility. So, what *is* the best way to start the conversation?

Conversation Starts with Relationship

Lay the foundation by building trust over time with consistent, compassionate conversations. Listen and learn what's important to the senior.

✶✶✶✶✶✶✶✶✶✶✶✶✶✶✶✶✶✶✶✶✶✶✶✶✶✶✶✶✶

In the last chapter, we met Mrs. Clarke and her daughter, Eva. The daughter had grown up running at her mother's heels and over the years, they had developed a close, loving relationship. Mom taught Eva about jazz and classical music. They took road trips, worked crossword puzzles, argued about politics, and generally hung out. Mrs. Clarke was very involved with Eva's husband and kids. She participated in Grandparents' Day at school and attended sporting events and other special activities. Eva's little boy, Myles, even suggested that Grandma get a job as a part-time lunchroom helper at his school. During their special moments together, Eva listened and learned what was important to her mom, and Mrs. Clarke often asked Eva's advice about financial matters. Their relationship laid the foundation for the responsibility with which Mrs. Clarke eventually trusted Eva.

✶✶✶✶✶✶✶✶✶✶✶✶✶✶✶✶✶✶✶✶✶✶✶✶✶✶✶✶✶

Trust won't materialize just because you have good intentions. When you share an open, loving, concerned relationship all along, trust will be there when you need it.

How to Start the Conversation

The most important thing is *not* to wait for an emergency when emotions are high and you feel pressured to make decisions. Always show interest about how your folks feel and what's important to them without harassing or expressing worry. Take advantage of stories in the news or from their friends to discuss later-life challenges. These may present opportunities to learn what your parents think about handling these issues for themselves.

When you are gentle and consistent over time, you should be able to explore the specifics of your parents' health and wishes about care, finances, housing, relationships, and other issues.

Be Gentle and Sincere in Offering Help

You might say: "I'd like to learn more about how to keep you feeling great, instead having so much stress like Mrs. Friend," or "So many seniors are getting ripped off. I don't want that to happen to you."

Then, ask to go with them to have their doctor, financial planner, banker, or accountant explain what you can do to help. Be proactive, patient and persistent. When that doesn't work, it doesn't hurt to be a little crafty.

Start with Generalities Before You Zero In

Seniors might find it less threatening if the discussion isn't directed at their specific situation. Go for broader relevance. For example, as soon as people reach legal age in their state, everyone should appoint someone who would make decisions on their behalf should they become disabled. In Illinois, that age is eighteen (except for the purchase and consumption of cigarettes and alcohol). I began those discussions with my kids when they turned eighteen and took it as an opportunity to raise the issue with the entire family. We discussed this type of planning as a rite of adult passage, like registering to vote. It was not about age, death, or dying.

Appeal to Their Power

Many in the current generation of seniors are used to being in control. They don't take lightly to giving that power away. You might want to say, "You don't want *me* making these decisions. If you want this to go right, you need to tell me what you want."

Don't Be Afraid to Use a Little Guilt

When you hear of another family struggling with end-of-life decisions or legal issues after a senior passes on, you might be able to leverage that situation to start discussions with your senior. I find that if parents will not make plans for their own benefit, many will do so to relieve their children.

You could say, "Isn't it a shame about Mrs. Church Member? I bet her kids feel awful that they didn't know about X soon enough to help. You wouldn't do that to me, would you?"

Get Your OWN House in Order

It's easier to start care planning conversations with your seniors if you are planning for yourself. Prepare your own essential documents: medical and financial powers of attorney, insurance policies, wills, funeral plans, and other important issues. Make sure your potential caregivers know how to find these documents and how to open your safe or safe deposit box. (If you don't want them to have access now, make sure they know how to contact your attorney).

Don't forget to review your finances and retirement plans with a financial professional at least yearly, and make decisions to support economic security in *your* golden years.

Keep your health information organized (See Bernie Ryan's binder later in this chapter) and build a strong relationship with your primary care professional to protect your health.

Invoke the Grandparent Superpower

If parents will do for their children what they will not do for themselves; they will do even more for their grandchildren. Let your seniors know what your doctor or financial advisor asked about your plans. You can share how uncomfortable you were about beginning the planning process *before* you tell them how much better you feel having done it. (Do you see how that might work?) Share the plans you've made to make caregiving easier for *your* kids. It might start a chain reaction that helps you as well.

Remember, Your Parents Are Adults

Unlike Chapter Three: *When The Doctor Says It's Not Safe for Them To...*, this chapter is about working with parents *before* they become ill. However, disabled or not, your parents don't become *children* when you want to help them. With your busy schedule, it might seem more convenient to rush in and take over. Maybe doing that makes you feel less fearful. Whether you do it for convenience or a sense of control, strong-arm tactics won't work. You didn't tell Mom what to do when you were little. She isn't going to take that well, today.

You're an Adult Too

Your parents are always Mom and Dad but by the time you are an adult, the relationship should be more mutual than it was when you were growing up.

You can't keep sitting in their laps or their pockets. Adult children who are emotionally and financially dependent on their parents have conflicts of interest that make them less capable of recognizing the seniors' problems. When you take full responsibility for yourself, you can be open to hearing, seeing, learning about, and considering your parents' concerns.

D'Nile Ain't Just a River in Egypt, Don't Deny the Need to Plan for Eldercare

It's easy to understand why pre-caregivers avoid thinking about eldercare. They're already dealing with relationships, childcare, student loans (theirs and their kids'!), other debt, jobs, politics, climate change, pandemics, and everything else. Many won't think about this topic because they are terrified of facing a time when Dad won't be around to support them (emotionally or financially). It can be worse to know that one day, Mom will still be here but won't be able to offer comfort, advice, or encouragement. Even if the relationship with your seniors wasn't great, it can still be hard to think about a time when they won't be the way you've grown accustomed to them.

Any of these fears can make caregivers deny the need to plan. Then, emergencies come and they are not prepared to give the care their seniors need.

Don't let "Ageism" Make You a Caregiver Before You Need to Be

Gray Panther founder, the late Maggie Kuhn, said "Age is not a disease." Ageism is a bias against older adults that causes discrimination in employment and other opportunities. Ageism is also an expectation that older adults should be disabled and just sit on porches and rock. This may make seniors and adult children accept disability rather than investigate possible treatment for changes in health and function. This can also make adult children rush into the caregiving role before the senior is disabled.

****

My Aunt Terri is ninety-three years old. After almost twenty years, she stopped teaching line-dancing classes at the senior center every week. Despite trying several different hearing aids, she could no longer hear the nuances of the music and decided she could not be an effective teacher. Even though her students disagreed, nothing has ever gotten between Aunt Terri and her decisions. She continued to drive to the center twice a week to dance and help plan the bus and train trips. She travels somewhere every couple of months and walks seventeen laps around a track in twenty minutes every day.

One spring, Aunt Terri said she felt too short of breath to complete more than ten laps. Several people said that was okay because she needed to "slow down" at her age. My response was, "She could do it a month ago; she was ninety-three-years-old then too." My cousins and I agreed with Aunt Terri that it was time for an appointment with her doctor. The day before the appointment, a hard rain caused the unusually high pollen counts to drop. She did her seventeen laps the next day. After heart and lung tests came back normal, Aunt Terri's doctor recommended inhaled allergy medicine to help her breathe when she needed it. Aunt Terri still does all seventeen laps every day.

****

Age is not a disease but neither is it optional. Though she decided to accommodate her hearing loss, my Aunt Terri would never have curtailed her activities without understanding why because she's "all that and a bag of chips!" Less intrepid seniors might just accept disability, not be willing to investigate, and set themselves on the downward spiral that occurs when people stop moving. Eventually, those seniors would need caregivers while Aunt Terri continues to be independent and maintains a quality of life she values.

It is not appropriate to burden seniors with tests that cause harm or more discomfort than the symptoms. Nor is it appropriate to subject them to tests that provide no information to support wellness. However, it is equally inappropriate to refuse to investigate a change in condition or behavior that might improve. Don't succumb to ageism and expect that seniors *should* be less capable.

Remember the LOCRx (See Chapter Three: *When the Doctor Says It is Not Safe for the Senior To... Balance Independence and Safety.*) Find out what the senior needs and make the appropriate response. Always ask yourself what you will do when they need more help. Then, plan. If you approach helping seniors in this way, you will not scramble to set up unnecessary, intrusive, or ineffective care plans. Neither will you miss opportunities to improve their health and quality of life. You will also have time to prepare for any changes.

I know you're busy. You fear losing them and your relationship with or image of them. Still, you need to prepare to do the job well. Keep your eyes open and keep an open mind as you watch for signs that your seniors might need help.

Do They Need Help? This Is What You're Looking For

In 2017, the Mayo Clinic website posted these alerts for problems.[46] Are your aging parents:

- Taking care of themselves?
- Experiencing memory loss?
- Safe in their homes?
- Safe on the road?
- Losing weight?
- In good spirits?
- Still social?
- Able to get around?

Although these questions are important, I recommend a few more specific questions.

- Do they seem to have more trouble with hearing or vision?
- Do they have repeated falls?
- Are they less concerned about hobbies and usual interests, appearance, hygiene, or housekeeping?
- Is there too little food or rotting food in the house?
- Are there dirty dishes, burned pots, or fewer pots (which may have been burned and discarded)?

Monitor Your Senior's Financial Health Too

Be suspicious if a senior begins to mismanage money.

- Does he pay bills late or forget to pay bills?
- Is she getting collection notices? (I'm not asking you to open their mail. Just keep your eyes open and ask.)
- Does he spend large amounts of money on strange purchases?
- Does she talk about contributing to lots of "charities?"
- Does he seem to have less money (refusing to purchase necessary items, saying he doesn't need them, or asking you to pay for them)?
- Do strange people call or hang around?

Watch Out for the Widowed

As we discussed in Chapter Four: *When Seniors Mismanage or Struggle with Money*, the death of a spouse can throw a previously comfortable senior into poverty. Income decreases (the total amount of retirement funds and Social Security income) while housing costs, taxes, house and car repairs don't usually change. Food and utility costs could decrease though the amount is not likely to offset the lost income. Medical expenses can threaten everything.

Don't Ignore Other People's Concerns

Your bossy sister, nosy brother-in-law, or busybody auntie might be annoying. That doesn't mean they are wrong. Even if you don't see a problem with your senior, others may have valid concerns. Take off the emotional blinders and consider all reports, carefully. Find a geriatrics program and get the LOCRx. That will let you know what, if anything you need to do.

Keep Information Organized with Bernie Ryan's Binder

Bernie is one of my Care Warriors. When her mom and dad were my patients, Bernie kept a medical information binder for each parent. It was a three-ring binder with section tabs and a specific place each type of health-related paperwork.

Bernie had several siblings, many of whom did not live in town (one was out of the country) Whenever a sibling helped Bernie by bringing the seniors to my office, the sister or brother had the binder. Although the visiting sibling wasn't the primary caregiver and might not have the most current information, the binder held the essentials. Bernie even had a section where she recorded her questions and any concerns she had gathered from other siblings.

These are the sections Bernie used. I have added explanations for each section and suggestions I have added to Bernie's list over the years.

1) *Contact information.*

Keep phone, fax numbers, and email information for *all* the senior's health professionals, as well as their pharmacy, home health agency, durable medical equipment company, and other community health resources.

Add a signed and witnessed letter that lists every family member, friend, and others who have the senior's permission to discuss heath information with the health professionals.

2) *Medical history*
List current and past health conditions. Include pregnancies, surgeries, other procedures, and all hospital stays.

3) *List of medicines*
Visit www.drcherylwoodson.com to get your copy of the medication list I recommend, to help you organize each medicine, how to use it, which doctor prescribed each medicine, and why.

Most medical practices send electronic prescriptions directly to your pharmacy. If you still receive paper prescriptions, keep them in this section, and don't forget to call for refills while you still have at least seven days of medicine. This will make sure the senior doesn't run out if there are delays at the pharmacy.

4) *Insurance paperwork*
Use this section to keep identification cards and orders for referrals, tests, and procedures. You should also keep letters from insurance companies that confirm (or deny) authorization for health services and the explanations of benefits (EOB). This document tells you the amount your insurance company has approved and how much you must pay.

5) *Advance Directives which may include*:

- A living will that gives directions for treatment decisions in life-and-death situations

- The power of attorney for health care (POA) allows a person to choose a trusted advocate to make medical decisions for her if she could not do it herself. With the POA, the person can also outline the circumstances under which she would consider life to still be worth living

- The POLST (Provider Orders for Life Sustaining Treatment) is a more comprehensive document that outlines the treatment options a person would consider and for how long. It also gives the person's wishes the same authority as a doctor's order.

6) *Communication section*
Here, Bernie wrote down her questions (and any questions from

her siblings) before each office visit. You can also use this section to record the answers and instructions.

I recommend two more sections.

7) *Test results*
This is especially important if you have seen another doctor who ordered tests your primary doctor may not have seen.

8) *Calendar*
In addition to appointments and the timing of tests, be sure to include your appointments and responsibilities to avoid scheduling conflicts.

Even Though It's Uncomfortable, You Have to Ask about *Everything*

Secrets are touchy, painful, and embarrassing, but they can be disastrous if you find yourself surprised in the middle of your grief. Make sure to ask about:

- Other relatives
- Another spouse
- Other children or dependents
- Other assets or debts
- Accounts
- Credit cards
- Expenses
- Inheritances
- Insurance policies
- Investments
- Liens
- Loans/ Mortgages
- Pensions
- Property
- Tax assessments

Know Your Senior's Wishes and Resources

The following list is not meant to be exhaustive. Consult legal and financial advisors to be sure you have all the information you need.

- Would she prefer to live in her own home with help or in a nursing facility? Are there financial resources to support her choice?

- Whom would he trust to manage his money? How would he like his advocate to manage the finances.? Has he competed the necessary documents? What protections are in place? (Consult a banker, financial planner or attorney)

- Keep a list of your senior's advisors. If you do not have power of attorney, ask the senior for written permission to speak with these consultants:

  - Attorneys

  - Accountants, financial planners, tax advisors, investment brokers

  - Bankers

  - Insurance agents

  - Realtors

  - Professionals who maintain other assets (auto mechanics, home maintenance companies, jewelers, art restorers, appraisers)

- Know the location of:

  - Bank accounts, trusts, retirement funds, other financial documents, and how to use them (either through joint accounts, POA for finance, or trust officers), safe combinations, or location of safe deposit box keys and access policies.

  - Funeral and burial arrangements

  - Insurance policies

  - Wills and trust documents

  - Lists of assets and expenses for the surviving spouse

  - Leases, mortgages, or titles to cars, real estate and other property

  - Lists, photos, and appraisals of other valuables (such as art, books, collections, and jewelry)

To avoid overwhelming everyone, most families will need several conversations over time.

Pull Your Team Together; Get Other Family Members on Board

Even though a senior has several children, usually, only one or two participate in caregiving. Everybody else sits back and breathes a sigh of relief as they spout excuses:

"She's the oldest." "He's a nurse." "She lives there." "He's not married." "She doesn't have kids." "He's the baby." "She has all that money."

Everyone has responsibilities that demand time, money, other resources, and energy. The siblings who live closest, don't work outside the home, are the most affluent, single, and child-free have as much right to their time, money, and lives as the rest of you. Even if the senior has specific expectations about who will give care, neither that nor other excuses gives the other family members a pass.

You're all family. Why would you want to kill one person? What would you do if the person you expect to give care couldn't do it? What if Big Sister died? Why increase that risk by leaving her alone in caregiving? Plan to work together now.

If you have been able to get your parents on board with care planning, their influence might pull your siblings together. Unfortunately, most families don't have that kind of luck. The primary caregiver must insist, and all the other siblings must realize that eldercare must be *fair*. It can be fair only when it's a team process.

It makes sense for nearby siblings to captain the care team and have power of attorney for health care; the people on the frontline *must* have authority to make decisions. However, the Internet, virtual meetings, and telephones make it possible for all siblings to participate from any location. Siblings with healthcare experience can participate in translating healthcare information, formulating appropriate questions, communicating with health professionals, and navigating the health system. Families can also benefit from the experience of relatives with legal or business backgrounds, and those with strong organizational skills. *Everyone* bears some responsibility.

The primary caregiver will need regular breaks and everybody can participate in the respite schedule. If you can't do a direct-care shift, can you provide transportation, pick up groceries, or prescriptions, help with laundry, cleaning, gardening, and visits to care facilities? You can also relieve the caregiver by picking up her dry cleaning, getting her oil changed, or helping with her children. Whether you're in or out of town, you can make phone calls to gather information, investigate care facilities online, help with paperwork, and contribute money to help with expenses.

In the ideal situation, the senior has already planned to fund their care.

Though this does not usually happen, adult children can begin the planning process in advance. Financial advice is a good idea at any age, especially in advance of a cash-draining situation. Offer to help your seniors find professionals to review their financial plan. You can also help them investigate long-term care (LTC) insurance options. My sister-in-law purchased her mother's LTC insurance policy twenty years ago and believes it was the best decision she ever made. Siblings can even pool resources to pay premiums.

Consult eldercare professionals, Area Agencies on Aging, Departments on Aging, faith-based eldercare resources, and other social service organizations. These professionals can guide you to programs that support seniors and caregivers. Get all the information you can to strengthen your family eldercare team.

"Teamwork Makes the Dream Work"(47)
...Until You Wake Up to the Reality of YOUR Family

When I was in practice, I hosted family eldercare conferences every week. Several of these meetings deteriorated into shouting matches that ripped open long-festering childhood scars.

"You're the favorite." "He let you get away with everything. "She bought you a car." "They always give you money."

These nasty feelings are disastrous for family relationships; they are also useless in providing excellent eldercare. *Get over it, get through it, or put it aside for now.* Once the caregiving season is over and you've given the best possible eldercare, you and your siblings can go into family therapy or go your separate ways. Right now, try to work together to get the job done.

Unfortunately, some families can't communicate, confront difficult topics, or even get along. Please see my book, *To Survive Caregiving: A Daughter's Experience, A Doctor's Advice,* the companion volume to this book. Chapter Five: *Don't Despair – There IS Help,* will give you specific information on ways to encourage communication and cooperation within your family. However, if you can't get help from your siblings, the community eldercare network will be your team (Departments on Aging, Area Agencies on Aging, and other resources).

Prepare to Take Care of Their Caregiver

This section should have been first. I didn't think you'd read it then. When you start your caregiving journey, like all battles, you must suit up first. Remember the fifth of my Five Keys to Caregiver Survival (See pg. viii).

5) Put Your Mask on First (This is what flight attendants tell you to do in case of an emergency).
You can't take care of them if you don't take care of YOU.

Your Physical Health

Go to www.drcherylwoodson.com and request the article on how to *Age Excellently* and the handout "You Should Know These Numbers Like You Know Your Social Security Number." These resources offer basic information about taking control of your health care and formulating questions to ask your primary care professional.

Your Financial Health

People can get car loans, mortgages, educational loans, business loans, and credit cards. *Adults can borrow money for everything in this country except being old.* Earlier in this book, we saw the financial dangers that can stalk seniors. Visit a financial planner to develop a budget, manage debt, review savings and investments, and make important adjustments now. This will support your financial security in retirement and save your children from facing some of the stress you fear in eldercare.

I have heard many television financial advisors say that many people in the younger generations may not do as well with their financial security as their parents have. Your children may not be able to help you financially as you age. You do not want to hurt them by setting up conflicting obligations: having to choose between you and their spouses, children, debts, dreams, or retirement plans. Prepare to take care of yourself or, at least, have money available if they have to take care of you. Talk to your kids! Decrease their stress by having the planning discussion I recommended you have with your parents earlier. Give your adult children a fighting chance to survive caregiving.

Your Emotional Health

Caregiving will add to life's other stressors: the breakneck speed of life, taxing or unsatisfying work, fears about unemployment, unappreciative clients, bosses, or employees, long hours, and little vacation time. There are also personal financial and health challenges, family drama, violence in our communities, and uncertainty in the political environment, the larger world, and the future. Start now and create a peaceful sanctuary in the midst of that craziness.

Start your day with peace. Don't check email, social media, or phone messages until you've taken time for deep breathing, prayer, meditation, stretching, or exercise. Then, eat something healthy before you look over your To Do list for the day. Confirm that you've listed the tasks and appointments in the most productive order. Although we may think multi-tasking makes us more efficient, it can make us lose focus, make mistakes, and become less effective.(48) If you can accomplish one or two things well every day, that's good enough.

Make sure at least one of your daily appointments is with yourself. Put yourself higher on the "To Do" list along with your most important tasks. Carve out a time and choose a place where you will regularly enjoy an activity for no reason other than it gives you joy. It doesn't have to be productive, and it does not have to take a lot of time.

****

For twelve years, I managed a solo-private practice, while raising active kids. Most of my patients were seniors, but many younger adults had several chronic illnesses. To keep me calm, productive, and sane, I took regular Taekwondo classes. Also, my nurse and right-hand woman, June, would arrange my schedule so I enjoyed regular joy-creating time. If only for ten or fifteen minutes, I could count on time to write fiction on most afternoons.

****

Commit to this "you" time and protect it. Unless there is a life-threatening circumstance, make sure everyone around you respects that time too.

If stress interferes with your sleep, appetite, health, mood, relationships, enjoyment of life, and ability to function at home and at work, admit that you *are* struggling. Find a counselor to help you pull everything together. You are too valuable to disappear into stress.

Spiritual Health; Attitude of Gratitude, Self-forgiveness, and Positivity

Your spirit will be healthier if you start by being grateful for what went well (or didn't go as badly as you feared). Take time to enjoy even the smallest success, *first*. Then, you can ask, "Why didn't that work? What could I have done differently? How can I avoid that outcome in the future?

Stop beating yourself up. So many people look back at a situation and immediately focus on what *didn't* work. They ruminate and relive the anger, embarrassment, failure, guilt, or injury. They share all that with others who often reflect back the emotions, usually in concentrated form. If you stew in that negativity, you can extend it into the future and miss opportunities for future improvement and happiness.

Dr. Cynthia T. Henderson is one of the most masterful administrators I've ever seen, and I was blessed to be part of her team at Oak Forest Hospital in the Chicago area. She taught me to ask, "What *can* work?" Many of us marinate in misery. We remember what went wrong, focus on what we can't do, and complain about the obstacles in our paths. Instead, we should identify resources and strategies so we can think our way out of tough spots.

Also remember the second of my Five Keys to Caregiver Survival (See pg. viii or request a copy of the list at www.drcherylwoodson.com).

> 2) Take the S off Your Chest or Step Away from the Kryptonite. You are not *Supercaregiver!*
> *You DO need help.*

You will *not* be able to anticipate every problem. You will *not* be able to prevent or resolve every challenge. You *will* make mistakes. Accept that and forgive yourself. Understand that you *cannot* do everything alone. Gather the necessary information; seek professional advice and *use* it. Look for opportunities to do better and give yourself credit for doing the best you can.

Stop Beating Up Others Remember, your seniors and other family members don't have "S" on their chests either. Forgive them. They can only do what they can (or will do). It takes a lot of energy to hold grudges. You need every bit of that energy to take care of your seniors, your other responsibilities, and yourself. In his life-changing book, *When Forgiveness Doesn't Make Sense*, Robert Jeffress[49] tells us that when we forgive, we free ourselves from emotions that sap our energy and destroy our joy. He emphasizes that forgiveness does not mean the situation is right or that you should keep people in your circle of trust when they disappoint or injure you. Forgiveness takes power from the people or situations that hurt you so you can handle your business and go on with your life.

Please see *To Survive Caregiving, A Daughter's Experience, A Doctor's Advice,* the companion to this book, Chapter Ten: *Get Help From Family and Friends,* for more effective ways to engage other potential eldercare team members. Also, look at Chapter Fourteen: *Protect Your Spiritual Health – Put on the Armor of Peace; Wield the Sword of Forgiveness* for more information about the power of forgiveness.

Preparing to care requires that you learn your seniors' wishes and collect the information you need be an outstanding eldercare advocate. Even with the best relationship, these difficult discussions require compassion, patience, and skill. The key is not to ignore or harass. Minister Gloria Randolph is the founder of Giving God the Glory Ministries (www. gggministries.com) Rev. Glo teaches that *the gift of PRESENCE is so much more important than PRESENTS.* Don't wait until there is an emergency. Invest in loving, trusting relationships now. Find out what is important to the people you love. Share activities you enjoy, use patience and gentle perseverance as you bring up eldercare planning issues during normal conversations. Stay alert. Commit for the long haul and know that you will make progress in baby steps.

While you're preparing to care for your seniors don't neglect your own physical, financial, emotional, and spiritual health. Leading by example can influence your seniors. This can also make it easier for your children to take care of you and themselves when the time comes. Above all, don't be afraid. There is a lot of help available to you. *You CAN do this.* The next chapter gives you information about how to enlist your professional care team.

CHAPTER 13

The Caregiver's Role in the New Healthcare System — You Are the Glue

The United States spends more money on health care per person and has more subspecialty doctors than any other nation, yet we rank thirty-seventh in the health of our citizens. We also rank near the bottom for health system efficiency.[50, 51, 52] All this money does not make up for a health system of disconnected towers of care: doctors' offices, clinics, home health agencies, emergency rooms, urgent care facilities, hospitals, assisted-living communities, and nursing homes. People move back and forth between care sites without effective communication between health professionals, patients, and families. Important information often falls through the cracks. Incomplete transfer of information between care sites can also lead doctors to misunderstand the care plan, repeat some tests, overlook others, fail to follow up on information found in other locations, and prescribe conflicting medicines. Health care professionals call this "fragmented care." Because of this disjointed system, the money we spend does not protect Americans from poor health, disability, and death.

An Example of a Failed System

****

In 1994, Lutheran General Hospital in the Chicago suburb of Park Ridge produced a film about Mrs. Dorothy Peterson. This vibrant, active senior moved through our health system and despite expert medical care, lost her health, her independence, and her life. Visit the Terra Nova Films website (www.terranova.org/film-catalog/mrs-dorothy-peterson-a-case-study) to find this resource.

The producers wrote this summary:

"Over the course of a two-month illness, Dorothy Peterson spent 38 days in the hospital. She was admitted, transferred, readmitted, transferred and readmitted in an out of various health care sites. She encountered caring and skilled staff but she also encountered a health care system where duplication of efforts and fragmentation of service frustrate patients and staff alike. During her relatively short illness, eight assessments and six nursing care plans were written."

****

Primary care physicians used to supervise their patients' health services in every care site and provide the coordinating memory throughout the system. In this age of shrinking payments and increasing administrative responsibilities, many doctors choose to focus their efforts in only one care site.

An increasing number of primary care doctors no longer see their patients in the hospital. In 2009, the American Board of Internal Medicine offered the first Certificate of Focus in Hospital Practice to "hospitalists." These doctors do not have outpatient practices; they are employees of the hospital or a company that supplies contracted services from doctors in many subspecialties. These doctors work only in the inpatient setting. Many hospitalists rotate on such a tight schedule that hospital patients can see a different doctor every day. This strategy confuses patients, families, and other healthcare professionals. It also threatens care coordination.

The Affordable Care Act

Our nation tried to undergo major changes to tame out-of-control healthcare costs and improve our health. No matter how you felt about

President Obama, the *intent* of the legislation was to move away from a fragmented system that reacts to disease, values technology in acute care settings, concentrates power in the hands of professionals, and pushes for cure at all cost. The program intended to favor well-coordinated, community-based programs that promote wellness, empower patients and families, and focus on quality of life.

The New Health Care Paradigm

PAST		AFFORDABLE CARE ACT
React to Disease	⟶	Promote Wellness
Institutions	⟶	Communities
Fragmented Care	⟶	Communication/ Coordinated Care
Professional Power	⟶	Empowered Clients
Futile Technology	⟶	Advance Directives/ Hospice/Pallative Care

"It's NOT what's the matter with them; it's what MATTERS to them."

Figure 3

The legislation that began this process is the Affordable Care Act, passed in 2010 and confirmed by the Supreme Court in 2012. Some aspects of the bill are already in place, (like extending parents' health insurance benefits to adult children until age twenty-six). Still, the future of this legislation is in question. and there are many challenges yet to face. I believe the primary goals of the Affordable Care Act were to:

- Extend health insurance coverage to more Americans.

- Increase access to preventive care by eliminating out-of-pocket costs for screening tests.

- Make insurance companies less restrictive about to whom they offer coverage and more accountable for their policies and coverage decisions.

- Identify and share information about models of care that provide better health at lower cost.

The new system intended to reward quality of care that promotes health, prevents illness, and avoids unnecessary hospital days. Also, instead of calculating payments based on the number of tests and procedures, the system intended to value more efficient use of health care resources. Patient satisfaction ratings were also supposed to translate into higher payments. The problem is, health professionals and health system administrators have not caught up.

Old Ways Die Hard

Despite the push for change to support health and avoid unnecessary use of health care resources, illness has made money in this country for so long; it is hard to change the attitudes and behavior of health care professionals or administrators. In the old system, payment to doctors and hospitals depended on the amount of care provided (the number of visits, tests, treatments, and days in the hospital). Though this "do more; get more" system was a big factor in driving up healthcare costs, many healthcare professionals are accustomed to this way of earning income. They fear reducing the number of hospital days, tests, and treatments.

Many health professionals still admit patients to the hospital or keep them there for non-urgent conditions and continue to order tests, procedures, and consultations that could have been performed in the community. The stated reasons are not usually financial. Health professionals do this to be "thorough" or to ensure that patients follow a care plan. Hospital administrators are used to focusing on the number of "bodies in beds" (census) or on decreasing the number of unused beds. They are sensitive to the penalties they incur when a patient needs to come back into the hospital for the same condition within thirty days. However, they become worried when intensive home care services in the community keep patients from coming back after day thirty-one. Neither has the new system removed barriers that affect patients, families, and health care professionals.

The Current System Causes Problems for Patients and Families

- **Challenges in health literacy** (the ability to understand health information and use it to make treatment decisions) may be due to developmental conditions, diseases of the brain, learning disorders, educational disparities, and the level of fluency in the primary language spoken at your care site. Even people without these challenges may find it difficult to understand each diagnosis, or the reasons for specific recommendations when they are ill, in pain, or worried about the health of a loved one.

- **Social determinants of healthcare** may affect how patients fill prescriptions, follow directions and keep appointments. These factors include health beliefs and challenges with employment, finances, housing, hunger, transportation, mobility, other physical or behavioral health concerns, substance abuse, childcare, eldercare, competing responsibilities, and exposure to criminal activity and violence.

- **Caregiver issues** can raise barriers to a person's health when support-people have their own challenges with cognition (brain function) or the social determinants of healthcare.

The Current System Causes Problems for Doctors and Hospitals

- **Limited discharge instructions** rarely include protocols that monitor changes in a person's condition and allow doctors to change care plans *before* people become so ill that they require emergency rooms or hospitals.

- **Lack of cultural competency training in care teams** leaves professionals without the skills and policies to consider the culture, language, values, and health beliefs of patients, families, and communities.

- **Health care professionals have little information about non-hospital services**. Most health care professional training occurs in hospitals. Few professionals understand the abilities and limitations of different levels of care and the capabilities of community resources. Because of this, they discharge people from the hospital to care sites that cannot meet their needs. For example, the emergency room staff may discharge someone to an assisted-living facility in the evening with a long list of new medicines or special instructions. They don't realize that there are no nurses in the evening to follow those orders and that pharmacy services may not be able to deliver new medicines to an assisted-living facility for several days.

  Most discharge teams are unaware of professional eldercare consultants, Departments on Aging, Area Agencies on Aging, health ministries in houses of worship, and other organizations that can help families explore options to strengthen the long-term community care plan.

- **Poor communication systems between care sites** are frustrating and dangerous. Different care sites can have separate electronic health records (EHR) that are incapable of communicating with each other. Instead of improving communication and efficiency, EHRs can waste time and decrease efficiency. This contributes to poor health, increased cost, and increased stress for health professionals. Most systems focus on codes for diagnoses and procedures and use standard templates. These rigid profiles do not allow health care professionals to record the critical thinking that proves services are medically necessary and qualify for insurance payments. This leads to unnecessary denials and lengthy appeal processes that can delay care, threaten health, and increase cost. It also leads to frustration when after patient-care, paperwork and inputting information into computers make workdays considerably longer.[53]

The Current System Causes Problems for Everyone

- **Poor communication** between patients, families, healthcare professionals, and care sites (hospitals, doctors' offices and clinics, outpatient medical services, home health agencies, nursing homes) leads to care plan errors and otherwise avoidable returns to hospitals after discharge.
- **The system still focuses on a list of conditions** instead of the combined impact of those illnesses on a person's health.
- **It still focuses on doing things TO people rather than FOR people.** Instead of providing enough financial support to address social barriers to health, improve communication, and focus on quality of life, the system still focuses on tests, procedures, and other technology,
- **There is still too little awareness of community-based health resources,** which could result in more efficient use of hospital days. Health professionals, insurance companies, and families need this information.

Will Things Get Better?

I don't think it will get better any time soon. Health-professional schools still teach the old disease-focused care plans. Though some training programs are beginning to encourage students in different health professions to study together, most programs train only one type of professional. We need to work together in teams to improve health, coordinate care, and control costs. Most patient-care education occurs in hospitals. Schools rarely introduce students to community care sites (home care, assisted-living, long-term care facilities, senior centers) to learn what care can and should be done without hospitals. Few schools introduce students to community health advocates, faith-based health resources, social service agencies, or other partners that can address the social determinants of care. Until the health professional and administrative schools develop new educational programs, even recent graduates will not understand how to work in the new system. I don't believe fully-equipped health care professionals or administrators will be in place for another ten or fifteen years. I'm probably being optimistic.

This Is What You Need to Do

While we wait for decisions on what our health care system will look like and until professionals and administrators are trained and onboard, caregivers *must* be the glue. You are the only constant advocate for your loved ones across all care sites. It is up to you to be the team quarterback. *You can do it!*

Keep Health Care Information Organized.

I described how to use Care Warrior, Bernie Ryan's, binder in Chapter Twelve: *Prepare to Care*. I recommend using this type of organizer to stay on top of health information for you, your family and your seniors. Tech savvy caregivers can input the information and pull it up on their smartphones.

In the Emergency Room and When You Go Into Any Care Site:

- *Bring Bernie Ryan's binder (or your electronic equivalent).*
- *Have several copies* of medicine lists, allergies, current and past illnesses and surgeries, doctors' contact information, and advance directives (living will, POA for health care, and/or POLST).

Trust me. If you have one copy and give it to the emergency room staff, the nurses and doctors upstairs in the hospital will probably never see it.

Even if you stay in the emergency room, when the shift changes, the new nurse or doctor may not have the first copy. I have almost never seen this information reach the nursing home, rehabilitation center, or home health agency after a hospital stay.

Instead of feeling frustrated about having to answer the same questions over and over, assume that these people will *not* have had any opportunity to talk to each other. Be ready to say, show, and give copies of the information again...and again.

Be sure to have the originally signed form of the POA *and* several copies. Though you may be asked to produce the original, only copies should leave your hands.

- *Write down the name and contact information for the* attending *physician, senior resident, or fellow.*

You may see a flurry of doctors (hospitalists, primary care physicians, and consultants). There may also be other health professionals at all levels of training from medical and surgical subspecialties, nursing, social work, behavioral health, and rehabilitation services., It can be hard to know "who's on first?" While patients and families believe all doctors in the hospital are "the doctor," there *is* a chain of command.

The *attending physician* is the main doctor in charge of the overall care plan however, in a university-affiliated teaching hospital, the attending is usually more involved in teaching than in direct care. In these hospitals, the *senior resident* will have the most complete, day-to-day information. For consulting physicians in teaching hospitals, subspecialty doctors-in-training are called *fellows*. Though they work under the supervision of the attending consultant, the fellow is usually the point person for care questions. Here are some common consultants:

- Cardiology (heart)
- Endocrinology (diabetes, thyroid, and other hormones)
- Gastroenterology (or GI, for the stomach, liver, and intestines)
- Gynecology (diseases of the female sexual and reproductive system)
- Hematology/oncology (or Heme/Onc-cancers and diseases of the blood)
- Infectious diseases (also called ID)
- Neurology (diseases of the brain and nervous system)

- Neuropsychology (PhDs who are expert in how the brain works.)
- Physiatry (Physical Medicine and Rehabilitation or PM&R, provides intensive, physical and functional rehabilitation programs, usually after discharge from a hospital. These services help people recover from especially complicated conditions including strokes and other brain injuries, severe arthritis, surgery on the spine or other joints, or any condition in which the muscles are damaged or weak. There are inpatient and outpatient PM & R programs.
- Psychiatry/psychology (behavioral and mental health)
- Rheumatology (illnesses that develop when the body's immune system attacks its own tissues: blood vessels, heart, joints, kidneys, muscles, nerves, or skin).
- Surgery-general surgeons perform most procedures. There are also surgical subspecialties:
  - Cardio-thoracic (heart, lungs, chest)
  - Neurosurgery (brain, nerves, back)
  - Orthopedics (bones and joints)
  - Podiatry (the foot and ankle)
  - Urology (the bladder, urinary system, and male sexual and reproductive organs)
  - Vascular (blood vessels)

You have the right to understand how every test, treatment, consultation, or surgery will improve or cure a condition, increase comfort, or support quality of life. Don't be nasty about it; just ask "How will this help her?"

At Discharge from Any Care Site

Whenever your loved one changes care site (home to hospital, hospital to nursing home or rehabilitation facility, any care site to the home):

- *Don't just show up to give your loved one a ride home.* You want to park and be in the room to hear the nurse give the discharge instructions. Ask questions and take notes.

- *Compare medicine lists whenever you move between care sites (care transition).* Do this every time to make sure there are no missing or duplicated medicines. Be sure you have the correct spelling of both the generic (chemical) and trade (advertising) names of each medicine. For example, acetaminophen is the generic name; the trade name is Tylenol. I don't care whether you can pronounce the names; correct spelling is key so you know if acetaminophen and Tylenol are both on the list. That way, you don't risk overdose by taking both medicines.

- *If the discharge medicine list is different from the one at home, ask:*

    - Which list should she follow? Do we just add the new medicines to the old list or do we change everything?

    - If some of the home medicines are not on the hospital list, should he take them or not?

    - If the medicines are the same and the doses (number of pills or milligrams) are different, which dose should she take?

- *Check whether your loved one needs additional tests, visits to other doctors, or other follow-up outside the hospital.* You need to know how soon and in what order to arrange each recommended test or visit. Ask the nurse for the names and contact information for each doctor and call to make appointments right away.

- *Ask for written disease-management information.* This will help you watch for changes that might mean your senior is getting sick again. These instructions tell you how often to check blood pressure, blood sugar, weight, breathing problems, pain, and other important measures. This information makes you a more effective partner with you doctor in avoiding emergencies.

Disease-management instructions also tell you what symptoms to report, which symptoms require an adjustment in medicine, and which are serious enough to warrant an immediate office visit or trip to the emergency room. For example, people with congestive heart failure should weigh themselves daily and get instructions about what their best weight is. They will need to know what to do if the weight changes by a specific number of pounds in a certain number of days or if there is a weight change several days in a row.

- *If your loved one uses equipment or receives special treatments in the hospital,* ask whether this will continue at home. If so, request training sessions *before* discharge. Also ask the staff to be sure the equipment and supplies will be in the home when your loved one gets there.

- *Ask for a home health referral* and get the agency's name and contact information if:

- You still have questions
- The discharge nurse cannot provide disease management information
- Your loved one has several conditions or
- The medicine list and instructions are complicated

Avoid Unnecessary Visits to the Emergency Room and Hospital

- *Get the prescriptions filled right away and talk to the pharmacist about any questions.* Remember, pharmacies search for the best prices on medicine and they may purchase medicines from different manufacturers every month. Each time you refill your prescription, even if the medicine and the dose are the same, the pill might look different. Be sure to check with the pharmacist. Remember, it's okay to tape a pill to the medicine list to help you identify the right one. Request a copy of the medication list I recommend at www.drcherylwoodson.com and read more about it in my book, *To Survive Caregiving: A Daughter's Experience, A Doctor's Advice*, the companion book to this volume.

- *If the doctor arranged a home health referral and you haven't heard from the agency within forty-eight hours* after discharge, call the agency. Ask the nurse for the number before you leave the hospital.

- *Make a follow up appointment with your doctor right away.*

Schedule All Recommended Doctor Appointments Right Away

Although subspecialists may schedule follow-up visits several weeks out, research shows that people are less likely to return to the hospital when they see the primary care professional soon after discharge.[54] Call for your primary care appointment right away and try to schedule the visit within seven to ten days. When you make your appointment:

- *Be sure the doctor's office staff knows that your loved one just got out of the hospital* and you want to make the follow-up visit as recommended in the discharge instructions. This may make it easier to get a timely appointment.

- *Ask if the doctor wants any tests or other information before the office visit.* If your health insurance plan requires referrals, arrange to pick them up or receive them by fax or secure email. (Don't wait for snail mail.)

- *Tell each doctor's office the approximate dates of your other appointments.* "My appointment with my Dr. A. is (DATE) and the doctor wants to see your results first. How soon can we get in?"

- *Prepare for the "Brown Bag" test.* Health care professionals call this the "brown bag" test because we ask families to empty all cabinets, drawers and other potential hiding places, find every medicine bottle, throw it in a brown paper bag (or some other container), and bring it to the office visit.

- *Bring* everything *to every doctor visit:* insurance cards, all the discharge instructions, medicine lists, your copy of Bernie Ryan's medical information binder, and copies of advance directives.

How to Work with Home Health Agencies

Medicare and other health insurance programs support "intermittent, skilled nursing" care for people who have had a change in their health. It must be possible to manage the person's needs in a couple of short visits per week (about thirty minutes each) over about six to eight weeks. *That's it!*

Because of decreasing insurance payments, some home health agencies offer services to healthy older adults. The agencies bill for the visits even though these people do not need skilled nursing services. Many seniors enjoy these visits and for many families, the extra visitors increase peace of mind. However, health insurance plans pay for skilled nursing services; they are not supposed to pay for friendly visits or supportive care. If agencies bill for non-skilled care, they commit fraud.

****

Mrs. Galloway was an active older adult, living in independent senior housing. She had a stroke five years ago and recovered completely. She had no care needs and was a safe driver. Her family was very loving and supportive, but their work schedules made it difficult to visit her until the weekend.

A home health nurse knocked on the door of Mrs. Galloway's apartment and asked if she would like someone to stop by from time to time. Mrs. Galloway agreed and enjoyed the nurse's visits twice each week until a physical therapist, occupational therapist, and a physician began to visit too.

In a routine office visit, Mrs. Galloway told me about these visits and said, "Doc, can't you get rid of these people? It seems like somebody's ringing my bell every five minutes."

The agency worked with a contracted physician and even though the nurses had an order from that doctor, these visits were inappropriate. Mrs. Galloway did not have medical needs that would have justified Medicare payments for these services. She did not have a new change in her health status. She was neither homebound nor in need of skilled nursing care. Even though my name was on all of Mrs. Galloway's prescription bottles, the agency never contacted me to help coordinate her care. This oversight increased her risk of drug interactions as well as unnecessary services.

I contacted the home health agency and introduced myself as Mrs. Galloway's primary care physician. I told them my patient did not need the services, that Medicare regulations did not allow for service delivery under those conditions and by billing for the services, the agency was committing fraud. The visits stopped. Mrs. Galloway and I discussed strategies to increase her social activities during the week and occupy more of her time until her family visited on weekends.

****

I realize that many seniors and families appreciate home care visits. Even so, these visits may not be eligible for coverage under Medicare and other insurance programs. Unless an older adult has experienced a change in her health that *requires short-term, intermittent care by a skilled nurse, nursing aide, social worker, or therapist,* use of Medicare funds for this purpose constitutes fraud.

While Medicare audits can result in fines and penalties for the home health agency, I am not aware that these costs are passed on to patients. Even so, exposure to extra tests and medicines are not in seniors' best interest. Also, why should the health care system waste money that can help people with *real* skilled needs?

If a home-health agency visits you, call your doctor. Also, give the agency your doctor's contact information. If the agency brings in a physician, contact your doctor and insist that the agency do the same. This will improve communication and avoid unnecessary tests or medication errors that cause illness from side effects or treatment. If your doctor agrees that there is a skilled nursing need, also ask for a social work visit to find assistance after the six to eight-week home health period has passed. If your doctor does not agree that you need skilled nursing, request a referral to a community eldercare agency to identify local programs to provide the services you need that health insurance does not cover.

More Organizational Strategies

You will need to be the information manager every time your loved one moves between care sites or interacts with any health care professional.

If you have a computer or smartphone (or access to them), it is easy to keep health information on a spreadsheet; print it out or download it. Be careful about using public computers and WiFi (for example in libraries) because people may be able to see your fainancial and personal health information. Many health systems have apps you can use to see your medical records on a smartphone If you search the Web for other organizational apps, be sure to check with your doctor and hospital about which ones are compatible with their electronic health record (EHR). No matter how you choose to record your information, update it at every care site and every time there is a change in medicine or condition. That way, you will be ready with current information no matter where your loved one comes into the health care system.

How to Manage Managed Care

The different types of health insurance plans create a confusing alphabet soup. There are HMOs (health maintenance organizations), PPOs (preferred provider organizations), POS (point of service plans), ACOs (accountable care organizations in which hospitals and doctors share responsibility for costs and care), and co-ops. There are also CCEs (community care entities) that coordinate non-medical services that affect access to care: transportation, prescription management, other social issues, and non-emergency health advice).

Most insurance plans have a deductible (an amount people pay out of pocket every year) before the insurance covers any costs. Depending on the policy, deductibles can reach several thousand dollars. Once the deductible is paid, there may still be co-payments: out of pocket costs due for any service. Some co-payments are flat dollar amounts, others are a percentage of the total charge.

In additional to traditional Medicare, there are supplemental insurance plans, and Medicare Part C plans with managed care partners. It is not always clear whether Medicare or the managed care or supplemental insurance has primary responsibility to pay for a specific service (like hospice care). This is especially true if the person has coverage from Medicare and an insurance plan from their job. It can also be confusing if the person receives services in the hospital as well as in outpatient settings. There are also plans for people who qualify for Medicare and Medicaid (dual-eligible), which adds another layer of confusion. The rules for Medicaid and Medicare change frequently and despite streamlined billing for dual-eligible patients, coverage questions can create nightmares for patients, families, and professionals.

What a maze! Most health care professionals have no idea how to help you navigate the system. It's hard for them to keep up with current regulations for every patient's insurance plan. Office staff, administrators, and billing companies may be equally clueless about rules. The person who purchased the policy has the primary responsibility to know what it covers, what it does not cover, and what paperwork it requires.

Understand the Policy You Purchased

It is important that you know the benefits of the policy, the exclusions, partial exclusions, and the level of your financial responsibility:

- What services does the policy cover and under what circumstances (Is there coverage for routine dental and eye care or only for oral and eye *surgery*?)

- Which services will the company decline? For example, will it cover elective or cosmetic surgery?

- If there is behavioral health coverage, does coverage extend to residential mental health and rehabilitation?

- Are there limits on the amount of service they provide in a specific time-period? How many days or visits does the policy allow per year?

- What are the deductibles, co-payments and maximum total payments allowed for each kind of care?

Get Help to Understand Your Policy

If the insurance company offers member information seminars, be sure to attend and read all the paperwork. If you still don't understand, employee benefits offices can provide information about employer-offered health insurance policies. AARP and Area Agencies on Aging can help you understand Medicare and Medicare Advantage and supplemental plans. State offices and community health advocacy programs can help with Medicaid questions. It is better to investigate before you decide where to have care. That way, you won't be surprised.

Understand "In-Network" and "Out-of-Network."

Most insurance plans contract with doctors in primary care, subspecialties, surgery, and behavioral health. The plans call these contracts "networks," and they also include specific hospitals, laboratories, x-ray facilities, and pharmacies. Your network depends on which primary care physician (PCP) you choose. Insurance companies will consider all other doctors and services "out-of-network." Even if a doctor, lab, hospital, or pharmacy has a contract with the insurer that issued your policy, if they are not in the same network as your PCP, your insurance plan will consider their services "out-of-network." Depending on the type of plan you purchase, the insurer will cover only a small percentage of out-of-network costs or none. Make sure that any doctor, care, or test site you see is in-network. Your PCP will have a list of in-network services and can help with this.

Be especially careful about emergency room visits and surgeries. Even if a hospital is in-network, the emergency room doctors, laboratory, x-ray, and facilities for surgery and other procedures at that hospital may not be. If the doctor you choose is in-network and that doctor works in several locations, be sure the site where you choose to have your procedure is in-network. It's best to investigate when you choose your insurance plan, PCP, and care site. That way, you won't be surprised by the bill for an emergency room visit, hospital stay, test, or procedure later.

If a required service is not available in network, the law requires that insurance companies pay for out-of-network care. However, they do not have to pay the entire amount the out-of-network doctor charges. You will be responsible for the difference between what the insurance agrees to pay and the actual cost.

Learn How to Jump Through the Hoops

- Referrals are orders for routine tests and consultations from in-network doctors. Insurance companies usually do not require referrals for emergency treatment. They do review requests for prior authorization. These cover requests for high-cost tests or treatments, special medicines, or procedures and wheelchairs, hospital beds, and other forms of durable medical equipment in advance.

- To improve the availability of common or routine services, most health plans generate a list of tests that do not require prior authorization. It is critical that your doctors become familiar with these lists and submit the proper paperwork when necessary. However, it may be hard for them to keep up with changes for every insurance plan. You can call your insurance company to see if the service your doctor recommends requires prior authorization.

- Some consulting doctors believe the PCP's referral covers prior authorization for all additional services. This is not true. The PCP referral covers the consultation only. If the consulting doctor wants to perform special tests or procedures, the consultant's office needs to contact the insurance company for prior authorization.- Insurance companies have a team of nurses and medical directors who determine whether requested services are medically necessary and whether they should be approved as inpatient or observation care in the hospital. These professionals also review requests for out-of-network care. This decision requires the ordering physician to submit medical records that show why the person needs the requested service. This is the information they need to give the insurance company:

  - What symptoms, conditions, or circumstances make the requested service appropriate (how do they affect the person's health, independence, or quality of life)?

  - What other (more conservative or less costly) services failed or were not appropriate for the condition?

  - How will the information from the test or procedure affect the person's condition (Cure? Decrease pain or risk? Provide information to guide the next appropriate test or treatment decision?)

If your health professional does not submit this essential information up front, your care can stall in a recurring cycle of denials and appeals. This can delay treatment and threaten your health. It can also cause you to pay large amounts for these services.

No Referral? No Visit!

Do not see any doctor or have any test or procedure without a referral unless you believe you have an emergency. The same applies to the many free-standing urgent care clinics. In life-threatening emergencies, you can get care without a referral or prior authorization. However, as I said, these situations are also subject to review. The insurance company's clinical team may decide that your condition was not an emergency and deny payment after you have received the service.

Know How to Handle Emergencies

Talk to your PCP about which symptoms she considers emergencies for your specific conditions. I taught my patients to call my office before heading to the emergency room unless they:

- Experience symptoms of a heart attack (which are often different for women)[55, 56]
- Experience symptoms of a stroke [57]
- Had a high fever of more than 103 degrees that would not come down
- Had seizures or were unable to stay awake, breathe, stand, or walk
- Were in uncontrollable pain
- Had uncontrolled bleeding, vomiting, diarrhea, urination, or
- Broke a bone and it was sticking through the skin

Also ask your doctor if urgent care is available in the office. In my practice, I set aside several appointments each day to accommodate people who needed to come in right away. Each doctor has a different threshold for handling urgent problems in the office. Make sure you understand your doctor's policy about which symptoms require an emergency room visit and how to receive urgent care in the office.

Don't forget that many insurance plans provide nurses who staff telephone hot-lines twenty-four hours a day. Call them if your doctor's office is not open, and you need urgent health care advice. You can also call if you don't have any of the symptoms I listed and aren't sure whether your problem is an emergency. However, *if you are afraid, don't wait.* Call 911 or go directly to the closest emergency room and have your family contact your PCP as soon as possible.

If the emergency room you choose is out-of-network, and the doctors decide you need come into the hospital, you or your family can avoid unexpected expenses by asking if your condition is stable enough for transfer to an in-network hospital. If not, the doctors who supervise your care will need to contact your insurance company and send records to document that the transfer was unsafe. Once your condition is no longer life-threatening, if you need additional hospital days, the doctors will arrange to move you to an in-network hospital.

It is up to you to advocate for your loved ones and avoid dangerous delays in getting the care they need, as well as unnecessary costs. Successful advocacy is an important job. It is also time consuming and can be very frustrating.

****

My daughter was under twenty-six-years-old and according to the Affordable Care Act, her father's HMOs covered her care. At age eighteen, she completed a power of attorney for health care document. I exercised it when she became gravely ill. When my daughter was well enough to move to a less intense level of care, though the health plan said this lower-cost service was a covered benefit, none of the in-network doctors specialized in the treatment she needed. As I said, the law requires insurance companies to pay for out-of-network care if companies offer a benefit and cannot provide that care in-network. However, the companies do *not* have to cover the entire cost; they don't have to do the legwork to find appropriate out-of-network doctors or guide those care teams through the prior authorization process.

My daughter and I requested the necessary referrals. The out-of-network care team submitted regularly updated information to document that the care was medically necessary. Even so, the health plan refused to cover services that the medical director and health plan administrators *had originally approved*. After what seemed like a million phone calls, emails, and letters, I was able to discover that there had been an administrative error: even though my daughter was the patient, the plan had begun to file all information in her father's name because he owned the policy. They had denied payment because there were no medical records in her dad's name!

****

It takes patience, organization, and perseverance to advocate for your loved ones in this complex health care system. Even so, *you can do it!* It's easier if you have executed health care powers of attorney before an illness. If not, you do not have legal right to personal health information and the insurance company will not have to work with you.

When a doctor orders a test or procedure, ask about referrals and prior authorization. It's best to be sure and call the company yourself if the doctor says these documents are not necessary. Encourage the doctor to send clinical information as soon as possible.

If the insurance company denies a service, the notice usually includes instructions about how to file an appeal. Ask your doctor to complete the appeal with detailed medical records to document that the requested service is medically necessary. It is important that your doctor does not send the same information for the appeal that she did prior to the denial. Your doctor can request a Peer-to-Peer discussion with an insurance company medical director who will explain the denial. This will help identify the additional information that is required for reconsideration.

Communicate with your doctors and insurance company in writing, and keep copies of everything. Use email and copy yourself, or use a delivery service method that confirms receipt. Also, even if your health plan approves a consulting doctor, please ask that doctor to send regular summaries of your care to your PCP. When you need more services than originally requested, ask the doctor to send the most current medical records to show what happened in the approved time, what they hope will happen in the additional time they request, and why other types of care will not work or could cause harm.

As I said, when necessary care is not available in the network, the law requires that the insurance companies approve out-of-network services. Despite the law, these out-of-network care encounters are not the norm. You will need to watch very closely. Clerical personnel often reject even fully-documented requests despite higher-level administrative approval. If you can't get help from the frontline, clerical staff, ask to speak to a supervisor. If you're still not satisfied, continue to ask to speak to someone higher up in the chain of command. Sometimes, it is possible to identify administrators and find their contact information from the plan's website. Communicate at the highest possible level. Keep copies of all medical records and correspondence so you can submit it again and again.

Don't give up, but BE NICE.

I don't pretend this will be easy. Doctors and office staff may take offense when you remind them of the rules. Sometimes, it seems like insurance companies want to drown you in paper and hope you will just go away. You have to stick it out. Remember, it is important to *always* be professional. You have greater impact when you are prepared, confident, and *polite*. You should not be loud and *never* be profane. You want people to respond to your message instead of discounting it because your delivery gives offense.

If your efforts fail, contact your state Department of Insurance for information about your rights, your insurance company's responsibilities, and the process for higher-level appeals.

Until the communications systems, professional education, and policies are in place to support necessary changes in the current health care system, *people will die.* Families need to stand in the gap.

You can do this!

CHAPTER 14

Wisdom from the Care Warriors

I convened several focus groups of seasoned, thoughtful, and very vocal caregivers whom I call the Care Warriors. I asked these women and several men to make sure I had addressed the right questions and had given complete, understandable answers. Several warriors watched my back by reviewing chapters. These intrepid caregivers also gave essential information and that wisdom deserves its own space. This chapter is that space.

I asked each group the same questions:

- What do you want to know about how to survive caregiving?

- As a veteran caregiver, what do you wish you'd known earlier in the caregiving process?

- What do you think new caregivers need to know right now?

- What were your biggest challenges (physical, financial, emotional, and other)?

- What impact has caregiving had on your life (short-term and long-term)?

- If you had one word to give caregivers, what would it be?

This is what the Care Warriors said.

You Have to Get Help

The main theme through all these focus groups was the importance of *not* trying to do this alone. These experienced caregivers recommended reaching out to family, friends, caregiver support groups, social service agencies, and clergy. They stressed the importance of maintaining strong social relationships to ensure that your life is about more than caregiving. (That means having fun and keeping up with your hobbies.) They emphasized the value of working with Geriatric Medicine specialists, and community eldercare resources like Departments on Aging, Area Agencies on Aging, and professional eldercare consultants.

Every one of the Care Warriors also recommended behavioral health counselors. Useless family conflicts and unhealthy behaviors survive because they've become familiar or comfortable, even for you. Although the senior and other relatives may not be up for family counseling, you cannot control them. You can control only yourself. Get counseling, and learn to give healthy, adult responses, even to the most frustrating, painful, and toxic situations. When people are locked in a dance and one person changes the steps, the dance *must* change. When you change how you respond, even if the other people don't change, the interaction has to change. It might not change the way you expected or wanted it to, but it *will* change. That gives you an opportunity to make new choices. Behavioral health counseling is critical for *you*.

Open Your Eyes

The Care Warriors believe you should be familiar with most signs of age-related problems and have a "what if" strategy. They agreed with the information in the Chapter Twelve: *Prepare to Care* and urge you to include health and social service professionals as well as attorneys and financial experts on your team.

It Is What It Is

I heard this phrase over and over in the focus groups. The Care Warriors wanted me to remind you of the commitment you made when you had your kids; despite PTA meetings, games, recitals, childhood illnesses and behavioral challenges, with some planning, you were still able to enjoy many activities and relationships. Eldercare is no different. Don't waste time grieving about what you used to be able to do, arguing with siblings, or feeling resentful. Do what you can do.

Care Warriors also said, "Your life, as you know it, is over." No matter what you expected, once you accept the caregiving role, eldercare will *always* be on your "To Do" list along with your other responsibilities. The Warriors stressed the need to give up fantasies about what *should* happen and who *should* help. They encourage you to accept what *is* happening, make your plans, get the help you need to get the job done, and enjoy your life.

Conserve Your Resources, Live from Your OVERFLOW, and Exercise the Power of "NO"

The Warriors agreed with my coach, Monique Caradine-Kitchens (www. innermillionare.com) who teaches several useful principles that empower women to find spiritual fulfillment, financial success, and the ability to live their dreams. One of her most powerful concepts is Overflow. Monique says the Universe has more than enough to meet our needs. When we recognize those gifts, are excellent stewards of them, and express gratitude for what we have, our "cup runneth over." (58). Monique says if we want to realize that abundance, we must be especially careful not to waste our time, talent, treasures, and energy. Instead, we should learn to make wise decisions about how to use, support, and grow these precious resources. When we protect and invest these assets wisely, the provision for our day-to-day activities will come from the OVERFLOW and leave a huge reserve of stress-free security for emergencies. It also gives us a supply from which we can help others without depleting ourselves.

I shared the OVERFLOW concept with the Care Warriors and they ran with it. They recommended that you keep your activities in the area of your strengths and get help for everything else. For example, if you can't manage money well, consult a financial advisor. If your brother is a better cook, ask him to make meals and freeze them. The Warriors also warned against becoming overcommitted just because you *are* good at something. Even if you are the best cook, conserve your energy, control the amount of time you spend cooking, and limit the number of meals you agree to provide. People won't die from a bowl of cereal or a sandwich and almost everyone can boil an egg.

Avoiding over-commitment requires making friends with the word "no." The Care Warriors agreed with what I heard the great jazz artist, Nina Simone, say in concert, "You can use up everything you've got trying to give everybody what they want." Don't overextend yourself. This is probably not the time to agree to chair that fundraising committee even if the activity gives you joy. If you need to be involved, can you participate without having the responsibility of running it? Can you identify trusted deputies and delegate? Set your ego aside and conserve your energy.

This Too Shall Pass

The Care Warriors said, "It is what it is, but your life will not always be like this." This crisis is not forever. Caregiving is not forever. Setting aside opportunities for leadership is not forever. Having to plan every step is not forever. There is life after caregiving, and the Warriors said you shouldn't wait to live some of that life *now*. Even though the Warriors encourage you to do something for yourself every day and plan regular respite time and vacations, they recognize how hard the job is.

Care Warriors Listed Specific Challenges

Physical Challenges

The Warriors cited sleep-deprivation as the number-one physical concern. Although they recognized having too little time to sleep as a problem, they thought the more pressing concern was being unable to turn off the worries and settle into sleep. They addressed the time factor by recruiting friends and family, using community services, hiring help, and planning rest time. They settled their minds by prayer, relaxing reading, and mind-body techniques like meditation, deep breathing, Yoga, and stretching. Many said daily exercise made it easier for them to fall asleep, though they found themselves "too pumped up" to sleep if they exercised right before bed.

Everyone advised against alcohol or sleep medicine, and I agree. Even though alcohol may make you sleepy, your body metabolizes it into compounds that make your sleep less restful. Sleep medicines may make you groggy the next day and lead to accidents and medication errors. They can also become addictive. Make sure to discuss options with your doctor.

The Care Warriors also reported back injuries and other musculoskeletal problems from lifting and moving adults with motor disabilities. The best way to avoid this is to be in the best possible shape. Start a regular exercise program with at least a few sessions with a certified personal trainer. This helps you improve core strength, posture, and overall fitness while avoiding injury. Physical therapists can teach body mechanics: the proper way to move people regardless of their size, weight, or ability to help you. Using joint position, gravity, the disabled person's body weight, and your own, therapists teach you how to use the least amount of energy to move people without injuring them or yourself.

Physical therapists can also recommend ways to improve safety, function, and mobility by changing the environment (for example, decreasing clutter and removing loose rugs, building ramps, and installing grab bars). Occupational therapists develop rehabilitation programs that increase a person's independence in performing activities of daily living like dressing, eating, and opening packages. These rehabilitation professionals can also teach you and your seniors how to use adaptive equipment safely (gait belts, canes and walkers, long-handled grabbers, modified knives, forks, and other items). Health insurance pays for these items when a health professional writes a prescription and documents that the equipment is medically necessary. If there are still out-of-pocket costs, long-term care insurance may cover some of it. Also, your financial advisor can tell you about possible tax benefits. Community health organizations may know about private grants, equipment donation centers, loaner programs, and other ways to fund these devices.

A rehabilitation professional should *prescribe* your assistive device. Please don't go into a drug store, big-box store, or even a medical supply store to buy a cane, walker, or other device without knowing the specific type of equipment that is best for your mobility challenge. Do you need a straight cane or a 4-pronged quad cane? Do you need a right-handed or left-handed quad cane? Is the cane the correct length for your height? These professionals have advanced degrees for a reason. Let them do the job for you.

Financial Challenges

The Care Warriors encourage you to find all the programs and financial resources that may be available for your senior. A professional eldercare consultant can point you in the right direction. Visit the Aging Life Care Association, (formerly The National Association of Professional Geriatric Care Managers) www.aginglifecare.org. Put in your senior's zip code to find a list of nationally certified eldercare consultants in or near that location. Local Departments on Aging and Area Agencies on Aging are other resources.

The Warriors were also worried about caregivers who retire early to give care without maximizing their retirement savings. The Care Warriors recommend getting thorough information as early as possible so you can make better decisions about investments and Social Security to ensure your own financial stability in retirement.

They recommended that you should be especially careful when you investigate the pros and cons of filing bankruptcy for seniors and yourself. For investment strategies and questions about bankruptcy, the advice of a certified financial planner is key. Remember to check with organizations like the Certified Financial Planner Board (www.cfp.net), National Foundation for Credit Counseling (www.nfcc.org), or the National Association of Personal Financial Advisors (www.napfa.org), to get information on professionals before you consider engaging their services.

The Warriors also urge you to keep detailed, thorough, and up-to-date financial records with separate documents for expenses paid with your senior's money and those that you pay out of your pocket. This is critical to avoid committing financial exploitation and for proof of appropriate use of funds should any questions arise.

Emotional Challenges

The Care Warriors know that you often feel angry with the senior, with God (for the faith-based,) or with yourselves. They said you may also feel deprived, as if you've lost yourself. Resentment is especially strong if you believe you are indulging or enabling seniors who aren't as sick as they say they are. This can be worse if you and your senior have unresolved disappointment, or conflict. However, *guilt* was the biggest emotional challenge the Warriors identified. While you are giving care, you can worry that your best isn't good enough. They understand that you feel guilty if you don't do absolutely everything for the senior. You can also feel selfish if you do *anything* for yourself. Even so, the Care Warriors said the most powerful guilt occurs when you feel relieved once the caregiving responsibility has passed.

Use the Guilt; Lose the Shame

In the first edition of *To Survive Caregiving*, I said guilt was a useless emotion. The Warriors helped me understand that guilt is not the problem; the destructive emotion is shame. They agree with Melody Beatty's explanation in her book, *Beyond Codependency*. She explains that guilt understands that what you did was either inappropriate or below the standard you wish you had met. Guilt gives you a chance to apologize, make it right, or change your actions to do better in the future.

Shame doesn't care whether your actions were right or wrong. Shame insists that *you* are wrong, bad, lazy, worthless, and a host of other negative descriptions that make you feel bad about yourself. While guilt can empower learning and improvement, shame produces nothing useful; it undermines your confidence and erodes your ability to do *anything* well.

Accept That You WILL Make Mistakes

The Care Warriors stressed the need to be kind to yourself, accept that you are human, and understand that you *will* make mistakes. You *will not* be able to do everything and many circumstances *will* be beyond your control. Acceptance resolves anger and fights shame. When things don't go well, forgive yourself and understand that the action is the problem, not *you*. Then, you can strategize about how to improve the action.

Acceptance Bursts the Negatives and Helps You "Keep it Movin'"

Over and over the Warriors expressed the need to accept what was happening and move on rather than be paralyzed by anger, complaining, grief, or guilt. So many times, during our meetings, the Care Warriors made statements like, "Yes, that happened. So, what do you need to do now?" "This is happening because of their decisions (or yours). So, what do you need to do now?" "That's not under your control. So, what *can* you do?"

They wanted to remind you that anger is a destructive energy-drain whether you direct it at yourself, other people, the situation, or at God. They encourage you to accept that you have *chosen* to give care; family members who don't help have chosen *not* to help, haven't they? You had the same choice but *decided* to step up.

The Warriors encourage you to let the anger go and accept that while it is difficult to shoulder this responsibility, you can learn to do the best possible job without destroying yourself.

Don't Risk What Is Most Valuable

The Care Warriors also remind you that *you* are your senior's most important resource. You take care of the senior's medicine, home, and money. Don't forget to take care of the resource that makes all this possible - your senior's caregiver. Hello, that's *you*! You deserve encouragement, support, acceptance, forgiveness, and a life. Some of the Warriors said they got sick because they forgot the F*ifth Key To Caregiver Survival: Put Your Mask on First - You Can't Take Care of Them if You Don't Take Care of YOU!* After recovering, they realized that it's not only okay for caregivers to take care of themselves, it is essential. They don't want you to make the same mistake.

They warn that if you do not address the emotional challenges that come with caregiving, you could succumb to self-destructive behaviors like overeating, overspending, and substance abuse. Many caregivers slide into depression. Some risk suicide. These veteran caregivers ask you to consult behavioral health professionals to help you work through your feelings and find ways to overcome them. They said, "We don't want you to lose your joy. You are valuable. We don't want to lose *you*."

Information Beats Panic

The Care Warriors suggest that you soothe anger, decrease frustration, drain guilt, and disarm shame by finding out exactly what the senior can and cannot do. As I said earlier, the LOCRx is a plan of care that geriatrics professionals develop. The professionals examine a senior's health status and ability to handle daily tasks. By explaining specifically what the senior needs, the geriatrics team will help you adjust your expectations and get organized to meet those needs. Once you know exactly what your senior needs and how to get it for her, you won't have to feel shame. You will be able to feel confident in your caregiving skills.

Spiritual Challenges

Several of the Warriors describe themselves as people of faith, and they say faith enabled them to overcome guilt, anger, and feelings of powerlessness. They report finding comfort in the belief that their struggles made sense as part of a larger plan.

The Care Warriors also recommended that instead of judging people, forgive and leave them to a Higher Power or their consciences. The Warriors urge you to redirect the energy you spend holding grudges toward taking care of your senior and yourself.

The Warriors want to make *sure* you forgive yourself. Use the LOCRx and the information in Chapter Thirteen: *The Caregiver's Role in the New Health Care System* to do the best you can. That's all anyone can expect of you. That's all you can expect of yourself.

The Short- and Long-term Impact of Caregiving

In the short-term, Care Warriors talked about sleep disturbances, physical ailments, and stress. They also talked about the strain caregiving can impose on a marriage because of conflicts over time, attention, privacy, and finances. Longer-term effects included the need to be needed, which may result in taking on more (and perhaps unnecessary) caregiving responsibilities in the future.

The Warriors also report a loss of innocence and trust. They described having difficulty trusting in people's willingness to help in caregiving but also in other situations. They said they had to overcome the feeling that if there was a good time, it could not possibly last. They recommend sharing these feelings with people you trust or with behavioral health professionals when you're not sure whom you can trust.

The Final Word According to Care Warriors

The Warriors say caregiving is all about change, most of which is unexpected. They agreed that flexibility, resilience, forgiveness, and a team are the most important factors in caregiver survival.

I heard Dr. Cynthia Henderson (the former CEO of Oak Forest Hospital, outside of Chicago) say "Blessed are the flexible for they shall not be bent out of shape."

"Resilience creates peace in the face of chaos," is one of the affirmations in my book *Dear Lauren, Love Mom: 31 Days of Affirmations for My Daughter, for Myself, and for YOU* that I wrote to encourage my daughter.

In one of my focus groups, Care Warrior, Kirk Riddle, quoted a counselor who told him, "To live is to change. To live well is to change frequently."

The Warriors agreed with Kirk, Dr. Henderson, and me. They said caregivers should expect the unexpected, roll with it, and always have a plan "B." When things don't work as you wish, don't give up. Forgive yourself, get up, call on your friends, family, and professional support teams, and get back in the game.

CONCLUSION

You Can Do This! You Can Also Help Other Caregivers Survive!

I know you are overwhelmed. Even so, please don't think that caregiving is impossible. It can't be; too many people are doing it. Caregiving is tough and so are you. You can do it, and you don't have to destroy yourself in the process.

In these pages, you have learned how to gather the tools you need to work through difficult decisions. You have learned to be objective and consider everyone's needs when deciding whether to share a residence with your senior. It can be tough to support a senior without either imposing on her by doing too much or doing too little and leaving him in danger. Even so, you now know how to get a Level of Care Prescription (LOCRx) and be confident that you are doing exactly what your senior needs. You have seen that when you understand that you and your seniors are adults, you can either ease emotional tension or manage it more comfortably. Calm, and respectful communication is essential to encourage fruitful conversations about finances and care planning. By developing mutually trusting relationships over time and by being patient and persistent, these conversations guide care decisions now, in the future, and at the end of life.

With deeper understanding of how to navigate our confusing health system, skills to organize the necessary paperwork, and more effective strategies for working with health professionals, you are a more powerful health advocate. You know how to ask the right questions, of the right people at every healthcare site. You also know how to implement Plan B (C, and the rest of the alphabet) when the answers you receive don't quite meet your needs.

The information about Alzheimer's disease and other dementias will give you more confidence in caring for loved ones who have one of these conditions. You understand that these brain problems are not part of normal aging; they are terminal illnesses (cause death). Because of this, you can act quickly to get the diagnosis, put safe care plans into place, and support everyone affected by these devastating diseases. You are especially sensitive to the needs of "Another Kind of Widow," the spouses of people with dementia.

You are also aware of the risks for elder abuse and neglect in caregivers and in older adults. You can also recognize the different forms of elder mistreatment when it occurs. With this information, you can feel confident in getting help for affected elders and their families.

Although we have focused on information that empowers you to care for your elders, I have also encouraged you to focus on your needs. We have reviewed how to protect yourself from the damage stress can do to your body. I have asked you to look at how you feel about caregiving, your reasons for caregiving, and how to manage your expectations of yourself, your seniors, and others. We have also looked at meeting your needs outside of caregiving so you can have a full, healthy life during the season of caregiving and once that season has passed,

Finally, you met my Care Warriors, caregivers from my practice and other areas of my life who shared wisdom based on years (in some cases decades) of experience in healthy caregiving.

Don't forget that you are also a Care Warrior with experience and information. Newer caregivers need to hear that wisdom. There are several ways to join the conversation. Share your questions and thoughts by joining caregiver communities online and in your city.

I'm still here to hear and help you. What other questions do you have? I need you to help me too. What topics would you like me to address? You are welcome to contact me through my website, www.drcherylwoodson. com, follow and comment on my blog, *Straight Talk with Dr. Cheryl,* and post questions. Although I will not be able to address every comment, I will cover the topics you recommend in future blogs, podcasts, and video discussions. Like and Follow the Dr. Cheryl Woodson Facebook page to learn about events where we can meet either virtually, or in person when we can. I'd love to hear your comments.

We're a team. We can get each other through this.

RESOURCES

Get a copy of these free materials from www.drcherylwoodson.com.

- *The Five Keys to Caregiver Survival*
- *Age Excellently! How to Be a Silver Fox*
- *You Know These Numbers Like You Know Your Social Security Number* (health screening tests to discuss with your doctor)
- Instructions for creating Bernie Ryan's Binder to organize personal health information
- Dr. Cheryl's Medication Management Form

BOOKS

Beattie, Melody, *Codependent No More: How to Stop Controlling Others and Start Caring for Yourself,* Hazelden, 2011

Cade, Eleanor. *Taking Care of Parents Who Didn't Take Care of You: Making Peace with Aging Parents,* Century City, MN: Hazeldon Publishing and Educational Services, 2009

CoDA, *Codependents Anonymous*, CoDA Resource Publishing, 1997

Evans, Jimmy. *Marriage on the Rock: God's Design for your Dream Marriage*, Skills for In-Law Relations, Number One, the Principle of Honor. Zondervan, Corporation Grand Rapids, MI 2005   Also 20th Anniversary Edition, MarriageToday, April 30, 2012

Gibran, Kahlil, *The Prophet*. 1923 New York, NY: Alfred Knopf, Inc., 2001

Greeson, Hochschild, A, Machungh, A, *The Second Shift: Working Families and the Revolution at Home*. Penguin Books (revised edition), January 31, 2012

Jeffress, Robert *When Forgiveness Doesn't Make Sense*. Colorado Springs, CO: Water Brook Press, 2013

Jones, Laurie Beth, *Jesus in Blue Jeans, A Practical Guide to Everyday Spirituality*. New York, NY: Hyperion, 2011.

Katie, Byron and Mitchell, Stephen, *Loving What Is: Four Questions That Can Change your Life*. Harmony, 2003

Mace, NL and Rabins, PV, *The 36-Hour Day A Family Guide to Caring for People Who Have Alzheimer's Disease, Related Dementias and Memory Loss*, 5th ed. Grand Central & Style, 2012

Meyer, Joyce, *Approval Addiction: Overcoming Your Need to Please Everyone*. FaithWords, Nashville, TN 2005

Miller, Alice. *The Drama of the Gifted Child: The Search for the True Self*. New York, NY: Basic Books, 2008

Peterson, B, *Jan's Story: A Love Lost to the Long Goodbye of Alzheimer's.*, Behler Publications; Second Printing edition (June 15, 2010)

Siegel, Bernie. *Love, Medicine & Miracles, Lessons Learned About Self-Healing from A Surgeon's Experience with Exceptional Patients*. William Morrow Paperbacks, 2011

Caregiving and Eldercare Information and Support Services

This list is for your information, in alphabetical order. I do not intend it to be exhaustive or to serve as an endorsement of any kind. You will need to do your homework before you contract for any services.

Aging Life Care Association (formerly the National Association of Professional Geriatric Care Managers, Inc.)
www.aginglifecare.org, (520) 881-8008

AARP www.aarp.org/health (search "Caregiver Support")
(888) OUR-AARP, (888) 687-2277

AARP Driver Safety Program, (888) 227-7669)

American Geriatrics Association (AGS)
www.americanGeriatrics.org, (212) 308-1414

American Medical Association (AMA)
www.ama-assn.org, (800) 621-8335

American Medical Association: Physician's Guide to Assessing and Counseling Older Drivers 2005

A Place for Mom
www.aplaceformom.com, (888) 704-7787

Caregiver Action Network
www.caregiveraction.org, (202) 772 5050

Eldercare Locator-Administration on Aging (AoA)
(800) 677-1116

Family Caregiver Alliance
www.caregiver.org, (800) 445-8106

The Leeza Gibbons Memory Foundation, Leeza's Care Connection.
www.leezascareconnection.org, (888) OK LEEZA, (888) 655-3392

Mrs. Dorothy Peterson: A Case Study, Lutheran General Health System
www.terranova.org, www.worldcat.org

National Adult Protective Services Association (NAPSA) and the National APS Resource Center
www.napsa-now.org, (217) 523-4431

National Alliance for Caregiving
www.caregiving.org

National Association of Area Agencies on Aging
www.n4a.org, (202) 872-0888

National Association of Elder Law Attorneys (NAELA)
www.naela.org

National Association of Personal Financial Advisors (NAPFA)
www.napfa.org, (847) 483-5400

National Center on Elder Abuse, Administration on Aging
www.ncoa.aoa.gov, (888) 500 3537 (ELDR)

National Council on Aging (NCOA)
www.ncoa.org, (202) 479-1200

National Foundation for Credit Counseling (NFCC)
www.nfcc.org, (800) 388 2227, En Español (800) 682-9832

National Patient Safety Association, "Ask Me 3"
www.npsa.org

Today'sCaregiver Magazine
www.caregiver.com

Organizations for Specific Health Conditions

These groups provide information, promote health, or support research and education about a specific illness.

Alzheimer's Association
www.alz.org, (800) 272-3900 (24-hr hotline)

American Cancer Society
www.cancer.org, (800) ACS-2345, (800) 227-2345

American Diabetes Association
www.diabetes.org, (800) DIABETES, (800) 342-2383

American Heart Association
www.heart.org, (800) AHA-USA1, (800) 242-8721

American Lung Association
www.lung.org, (800) LUNGUSA, (800) 586-4872

American Stroke Association
www.strokeassociation.org, (888) 4 STROKE, (888) 474-7653

Arthritis Foundation
www.arthritis.org, (800) 568-4045

National Kidney Foundation
www.kidney.org, (855) NKF-CARES, (855) 653-2273

National Multiple Sclerosis Society
www.nationalmssociety.org, (800) FIGHT MS, (800) 344-4867

National Osteoporosis Foundation
www.nof.org, (800) 231-4222

National Parkinson Foundation
www.parkinson.org, (800) 4PD-INFO

National Stroke Association
www.stroke.org, (800) STROKES, (800) 787-6537

REFERENCES

1. American Psychological Association, Stress Effects on the Body, www.apa.org/helpcenter/stress-body.aspx, 2018 (accessed 21 Aug 18)

2. Harvard Health Publishing, Harvard Medical School, "Understanding the stress response: Chronic Activation of this Survival Mechanism Impairs Health" https://www.health.harvard.edu/staying-healthy/understanding-the-stress-response, March 2011, updated 1 May 18, (accessed 21 Aug 18)

3. Schwartz, M, "Robert Sapolsky discusses physiological effects of stress. Stanford Report, March 7, 2007, news.stanford.news.2007// March 7// S (accessed 9 Sept 2013, reviewed 21 Aug 18)

4. Ibid.

5. Centers for Disease Control and Prevention, Sleep and sleep Disorders, https://www.cdc.gov/sleep/about_sleep/chronic_disease.html 2018, (accessed 21 August 2018)

6. Colten, HR, Altevogt, BM ed. Sleep Disorders and Deprivation: An Unmet Health Problem. In National Academies of Science Engineering and Medicine Committee on Sleep Medicine and Research, National Academies Press, 1 edition, 14 April 2006 www.nationalacademies.org/hmd/~/media/Files/Report%20Files/2006/Sleep-Disorders-and-Sleep-Deprivation-An-Unmet-Public-Health-Problem/Sleepforweb.pdf (accessed 21 August 2018)

7. Ibid, Harvard Health Publishing

8. Post-Traumatic Stress Disorder, www.nimh.nih.gov/health/topics/post-traumatic-stress-disorder-PTSD/index.shtml May, 2019 (accessed 13 July 2019)

9. Byron Katie <www.thework.com/thework.asp >) (accessed) 8 August 2013.(reviewed 21 Aug 18)

10. Ibid

11. Byron Katie, *Loving What Is: Four Questions That Can Change Your Life.* Harmony 1st edition, 2003

12. Evans, J, *Marriage on the Rock: God's Design for your Dream Marriage,* Skills for In-Law Relations, Number One, the Principle of Honor. Zondervan, Corporation Grand Rapids, MI 2005 267-6

13. Exodus 20:12 The Holy Bible, KJV

14. Ephesians 6:1 The Holy Bible, KJV

15. Institute for Highway Safety, Highway Loss Data Institute, "Older Drivers" May 2018 www.iihs.org/iihs/topics/t/older-drivers/qanda (accessed 6 June 2018)

16. Ibid

17. Id. Colten, HR, Altevogt, BM

18. Adams, J, *When Our Grown Kids Disappoint Us: Letting Go of Their Problems, Loving Them Anyway and Getting On With Our Lives.* Free Press, 2004

19. Meyer, Joyce, *Approval Addiction: Overcoming Your Need to Please Everybody,* Faith Words, 2005

20. Codependents Anonymous, *The CoDA Book,* CoDA Resources Publishing, 1st ed., 2012

21. Ibid

22. Beattie, Melody, *Codependent No More: How to Stop Controlling Others and Start Caring for Yourself,* Hazledon, 1986

23. Alzheimer's Association, 2019 Alzheimer's Disease Facts and Figures Report, Alzheimer's Dement 2019 15 (3) 321-87

24. Anderson, Pauline, "Delirium Linked to Death and other Poor Outcomes in Elderly," https://www.medscape.com/viewarticle/726248, May 2010 (accessed 12 July 18)

25. Collier, R, "Hospital-Induced Delirium Hits Hard" CMJA 2012 January 10; 184(1), 23-24, on https://www.ncbi/nml/nih.gov/pmc/

articles/PMC32.pdf accessed) 20 August 2013 reviewed 8 Aug 18)

26. Gross, AL, Jones, RN et al, "Delirium and Long-term Cognitive Trajectory Among Persons With Dementia," Arch Intern Med 2012 172 (12) 1324-31 on <archin.jamanetwork.pdf > (accessed 20 August 2013 reviewed 8 August 2018)

27. Suicide Prevention Resource Center, "Suicide Statistics" https://afsp.org/about-suicide/suicide-statistics/2016 (accessed 26 July 18)

28. Segura, M, "The Other Half of the Story," *Sports Illustrated*, 117 (10), September 10, 2012 Reviewed 12 August 2018

29. Mendez F, "What is the Relationship of Traumatic Brain Injury to Dementia?" J Alzheimer's Dis. 2017;57 (3): 667-81. Doi:10.3233/JAD-161002, (accessed from PubMed.gov US National Library of Medicine, National Institutes of health https://www.ncbi.nlm.nih.gov/pubmed/28269777, 13 August 2018)

30. Ibid, Mendez

31. 2017 Profile of Older Americans, Administration for Community Living, Administration on Aging, April 2018, https://acl.gov/sites/default/files/Aging%20and%20Disability%20in%20America/2017OlderAmericansProfile.pdf

32. National Institutes of Mental Health, "Seasonal Affective Disorder," www.nimh.nih.gov/health/topics/seasonal-affective-disorder/index.shtmlNovember 13, 2014, updated March 2016, (accessed 17 August 2018)

33. Katz, S, Down, DT, Cash, HR, et al, "Progress in the Development of an Index of ADL, Gerontologist 10: 20-30, 1970

34. LaPook, J, CBS NEWS, 20/20, Following a Couple from the Diagnosis to the Final Stages of Alzheimer's Disease, 2008-2018, April 22, 2018 www.google.com/amp/s/www.cbsnews.com/amp/news/alzheimers-disease-following-a-couple-from-diagnosis-to-the-final-stages (accessed July 18, 2018)

35. Volokh, Eugene, 78-Year-Old Iowa Legislator Prosecuted for Having Sex with his Wife, Who Was Suffering From Alzheimer's Disease, The Washington Post, December 11, 2014, (accessed 7 February, 2015 reviewed 9 August 2018)

36. Resident population of the United States by sex and age as of July 2018 (in millions) www.statistica.com/statistics/241488/population-of-the-US-by-sex-and-age (accessed 8 March 2019)

37. Peterson, Barry, Jan's Story: Love Lost to the Long Goodbye of Alzheimer's, Behler Publications, 15 June 2010

38. Dialectical definition www.google.com/search/dialectical+definition/ (accessed 19April 2019)

39. Away From Her, Director-Sarah Polley, starring Julie Christie, Gordin Pisent, Capri Releasing, Echo Lake Productions, Foundry Films, Hanway Films, The Film Farm, 2007

40. Justice Not Jealous About Husband's Romance, www.nbcnews.com/id21773097/ns/us_news/life/t/x/ex-justicenotjealousabouthusband'sromance 13 November 2007, (originally accessed 13 June 2013, reviewed 28 June 2018)

41. "Mickey Rooney Claims Elder Abuse: Actor's Testimony to Congress Helps Spur Bill for New Crackdown," AARP Bulletin, March 2, 2011, <www.aarp.org > (originally accessed July 10, 2015, reviewed 8 July 2018)

42. Centers for Disease Control and Prevention, "Understanding Elder Abuse www.cdc.gov/violenceprevention/pdf/em-factsheet-a.pdf, May 17, 2018 (accessed 14 July 18)

43. Bowes, H, Domestic violence "grown old": the unseen victims of prolonged abuse, The Conversation, www.theconversation.com/domestic-violence-grown-old-the-unseen-victims-of-prolonged-abuse-43014 June 15, 2015 (accessed 12 Aug 2018)

44. National Adult Protective Services Association, Get Informed, www.napsa-now.org/get-informed/ (accessed 17 June 2018)

45. Wang, X, Elder Abuse: An Approach to Identification, Assessment and Intervention, https://www.ncbi.nim.nih.gov>pmc>articlesPMC4435869, 19 May 2015 (accessed 23 August 2018)

46. Aging Parents: 8 Warning Signs of Health Problems." https://www.mayoclinic.org/healthy-lifestyle/caregivers/in-depth/aging-parents/art-20044126 , 13 December 2017 (accessed 8 August 2018)

47. Quote from John C. Marshall

48. Skaugset LM[1], Farrell S[2], Carney M[3], Wolff M[3], Santen SA[3], Perry M[3], Cico SJ[4] Can You Multitask? Evidence and Limitations of Task Switching and Multitasking in Emergency Medicine. Ann Emerg Med. 2016 Aug;68(2):189-95. doi: 10.1016/j.annemergmed.2015.10.003. Epub 2015 Nov 14. https://www.ncbi.

nlm.nih.gov/pubmed/26585046

49. Jeffress, R. *When Forgiveness Doesn't Make Sense.* Colorado Springs, CO: Water Brook Press, 2008.

50. NPR Goats and Soda, Which Country Spends the Most (And Least) on Health Care Per Person. https://www.npr.org/sections/goatsandsoda/2017/04/20/524774195/what-country-spends-the-most-and-least-on-health-care-per-person (accessed 1 August 2018)

51. Murray, C.J.L. Phill, D, Frenk, J., Ranking 37th- Measuring Performance in the US Health Care System N Engl J Med 2010; 362:98-99, DOI: 10.1056/NEJMp0910064January 14, www.nejm.org/doi/full/10.1056/NEJMp09100642010 (accessed 1 August 2018)

52. Ellison, A, US Healthcare Ranks 50th out of 55 Countries for Efficiency, Beckers Hospital CFO Report, Financial Management, September 29, 2016, https://www.beckershospitalreview.com/finance/us-healthcare-system-ranks-50th-out-of-55-countries-for-efficiency.html (accessed 1 August 2018)

53. Kane, L, Medscape Physician Compensation Report, Pg 9 Medscape.com/Slideshow/2019-compensation-overview-10 April 2019 (accessed 5 June 2019)

54. DeLia D,Tong J, Gaboda,D and Casalino, LP. Post-Discharge Follow-Up Visits and Hospital Utilization by Medicare Patients, 2007–2010, Medicare and Medicaid Research Review, 2014 4:2 https://www.cms.gov/mmrr/Downloads/MMRR2014_004_02_a01.pdf (accessed 2 August 2018)

55. Mayo Clinic Staff, Diseases and Conditions www.mayoclinic.org/diseases-conditions/heart-attack/basics/symptoms/CON-20019520, May 30, 2018 (accessed 11 July 2018)

56. American Heart Association, Heart Attack in Women www.heart.org/HEARTORG/Conditions/HeartAttack/WarningSignsofaHeartAttack/Heart-Attack-Symptoms-in-Women_UCM_436448_Article.jsp, August 21, 2015 Accessed, September 22 2015 reviewed 14 August 2018)

57. American Heart Association, American Stroke Association," FAST : One of the Most Powerful 4-Letter Words," www.strokeassociation.org/STROKEORG/WarningSigns/Stroke-Warning-Signs-and-Symptoms_UCM_308528_SubHomePage.jsp (accessed 11 July 18)

58. Psalm 24:5 The Holy Bible, KJV

ACKNOWLEDGMENTS

In addition to my Father and my family, so many people have blessed me with their support. They encouraged, consoled, and cajoled me through my writing process. I especially want to thank:

- The editors and proofreaders who contributed to this project over the years: Joy Shields of Writer's Beacon, Liz Ridley The Writer's Midwife, Brittiany Koren of Written Dreams, my sister-in-law Brackette F. Williams, PhD, my cuz, Deborah Bennie, and my daughter Lauren Murff

- Mirella Tovar of Me Too Designs for the front cover and L. Julie Torrey Parker for the back-cover designs

- My coach, Monique Caradine-Kitchens and her life-changing conference, Overflow 2014

- Kathryn Kraynick, who helped me realize that this book was separate from *To Survive Caregiving: A Daughter's Experience, A Doctor's Advice.*

- John D from Codependents Anonymous

There are no words strong enough to fully express my gratitude for the Care Warriors who gave me their time, wisdom, and encouragement.

- Donna Brumfield
- Belinda Cannon

- Dana Davis
- Marge Foley
- Roberta Hartley
- Melodee Leimnetzer
- Reverend Ruby Meyers and her sisters: Dora, Romona, Regina, and Ellah
- Kirk Riddle
- Bernie Ryan
- Pastor Mike and Mrs. Debra Russell
- Joy Shields
- Kitty Watson and
- All the caregivers who shared their families with me when I was in practice. Thank you for continuing to support me at each of my presentations, and for liking and following me on social media, and connecting with me through my website, https://www.drcherylwoodson.com.

I am honored and so very grateful to all of you for blessing me and trusting me with your seniors, your questions, your stories, and your wisdom.

CW

Meet the Author

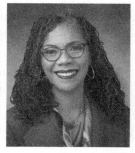

Dr. Cheryl Woodson has spent almost 40 years teaching and practicing Geriatric Medicine while raising a family and navigating her mother's ten-year journey with Alzheimer's disease. Dr. Cheryl offers a unique perspective: a professional's expertise tempered by a daughter's practical understanding and plain language. An informative, inspiring, and entertaining speaker whom the New York Times called "a blunt and funny woman," Dr. Cheryl shoots from the hip and from the heart to support family caregivers and the professionals who counsel them to give excellent eldercare without destroying their own health, finances, and relationships. She has also broadened her message to empower all adults move into the second half of life ready to *Live Out Loud & Age Excellently!* For more information, to learn about new publications and events, and to schedule a presentation, visit www.drcherylwoodson.com, follow Dr. Cheryl's blog, Straight Talk with Dr. Cheryl, watch her YouTube channel, and follow her on Facebook, Instagram, and TikTok.

Made in the USA
Middletown, DE
17 May 2023